Ambulance Mental Health Response

Terry Simpson

Printing history

This edition first published 2022

The authors and publisher welcome feedback from the users of this book. Please contact the publisher:

Class Professional Publishing, The Exchange, Express Park, Bristol Road, Bridgwater TA6 4RR

Telephone: 01278 427 826

Email: info@class.co.uk

www.classprofessional.co.uk

Class Professional Publishing is an imprint of Class Publishing Ltd

A CIP catalogue record for this book is available from the British Library

Paperback ISBN: 9781859599662

eBook ISBN: 9781859599815

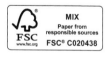
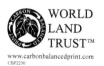

Cover design by Hybert Design Limited, UK

Designed and typeset by Fresh Communications and PHi Business Solutions

Printed in UK by Hobbs

Contents

About the Author

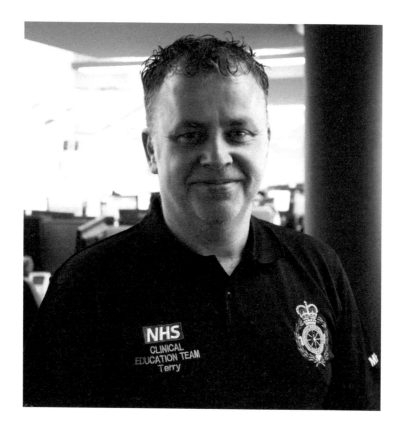

Terry Simpson, who currently works in an urgent and emergency mental health care NHS strategic transformation role, began his career as a mental health nurse 22 years ago. Working nationally across the ambulance sector, Terry was previously a Mental Health Lead at South Central Ambulance Service NHS Trust. With a background in adult mental health and crisis resolution teams, Terry also has extensive experience in education, patient care and improving ambulance mental health crisis response plans.

Terry joined the ambulance service wanting to improve patient experience, pathways, collaboration and joined-up services for patients presenting in crisis. He feels passionately that anyone in mental health crisis should have equal access to urgent and emergency care in a way comparable to any medical life-threatening emergency. Terry believes it is crucial to recognise that, like physical health, we all have mental health and consequently mental health is everybody's consideration.

Acknowledgements

The author would like to thank the following people for their involvement and support with the text:

- South Central Ambulance Service, with a particular thank you to Ian Teague, for their support in bringing about this publication.

- Elizabeth Biggs – Public Health Principal and Suicide Prevention Lead

- Alf Douglas – Creative Director, Fresh Communications

- Stephen Down – Mental Health Education Transformation Specialist and Mental Health Lead, NWAS

- Darren Earley – Specialist Paramedic

- Mairi Evans – Systemic Psychotherapist, CYPF and BEDS Clinical Director and Neurodiversity Lead, Berkshire NHS Foundation Trust

- Jules Fox – Approved Mental Health Professional Lead, Oxfordshire

- Chloe Lofthouse-Jones – Ambulance Dementia Education Lead

- Sonya McLean – Senior Transformation Manager for Mental Health Crisis Care, Hampshire and Isle of Wight ICS

- Reuben Pearce – Mental Health Nuse Consultant, Berkishire

- Georgia Pickwick – Mental Health Lead, Thames Valley Police

- Simon Tarrant – Autism and Crisis Care Pathway Development Manager, Buckinghamshire, Oxfordshire and Berkshire West Integrated Care Board

- Jaimee Wylam – Specialty Registrar in Public Health.

Thank you also to all the patients and carers with lived experience as part of the expert reference groups. Your contributions to improving awareness and education will help shape equality of access to emergency care between medical and mental health care. Whilst we may not have experienced the distress and trauma a mental health crisis can bring or impact on an individual's life, we can provide empathy, dignity and respect.

Class Professional Publishing would like to thank and acknowledge the following:

- All the anonymous reviewers who commented on earlier drafts of the text.

- Association of Ambulance Chief Executives for kind permission to reproduce the Mental Health Continuum on p. 95.

- South Western Ambulance Service NHS Foundation Trust for kind permission to reproduce the photograph on p. 11.

- Photos provided by Shutterstock (p.33 © eggeegg/Shutterstock; p.55 © Andrey Popov/Shutterstock; p.60 © Pkpix / Shutterstock; p.92 © SpeedKingz / Shutterstock).

- Photos provided by iStock (p.50, p.56 © SDI Productions/iStock).

- All other photographs and artwork have been provided by Fresh Communications and PHi.

Introduction

About this book

The purpose of this book is to give you an introduction and practical guide to mental health and mental illness from an urgent and emergency service perspective. Although the guide is far from comprehensive, it provides a broad introduction into common mental health themes for those working in prehospital care. There are sections which cover basic principles of assessment and treatment, as well as a glossary of commonly encountered mental illnesses. We have also included a section which examines the interface between mental health, mental capacity and the legal framework to support compassionate care, decision making, safety and proportionate risk management.

Responding to mental health crisis in the ambulance service

Mental health difficulties are unfortunately common, and one in four people will be suffering from a mental health problem at any one time. Responding to mental health crisis in the ambulance service can be one of the most challenging incidents you may face. Historically there have been gaps around collaborations between the ambulance service, police, mental health providers and approved mental health professionals (AMHPs) within social care.

AMHPs are responsible for co-ordinating Mental Health Act assessments. Referrals should be considered if a patient is refusing treatment and presents as a high risk to themselves or others in the context of a mental health condition. AMHPs work within social services and can be accessed for support via local operational contact details. Further details on legislation and support are provided on pages 34–40.

During your career you will be responding to patients presenting with mental illness. As part of the NHS long-term plan for ambulance mental health investment standards, ambulance services are building partnership-provider processes to support commissioner-led system transformation. Often the complexity of mental health conditions makes it very difficult for you to be able to work out exactly what is wrong or how you can assist someone in a crisis. You also may feel that you do not have the necessary skills to be able to assist someone in need, which is not an unusual feeling for many clinicians. The key principle is to have a compassionate, non-judgemental approach. Whilst we feel that on the whole our profession plays an excellent role in the early management of these patients, we also recognise that current training, support and development strategies need to be enhanced. In recognition of the significant role the ambulance service plays in responding to mental health calls, there will be a dedicated national investment programme to improve the capacity of the ambulance service to meet mental health needs (NHS England, 2021).

Your ambulance trust or employer may well have a database of services and signposting options, of which mental health pathways may be a referral route for support.

Part 1

Understanding and Assessing Mental Health

This section includes:

- **What Are Mental Health and Mental Illness?**

- **Causes of Mental Illness**

- **Initial Assessment of Patients with Mental Illness**

- **Dynamic Risk Assessment and Management Plans**

- **Legal Framework and Decision Making**

What Are Mental Health and Mental Illness?

Mental health difficulties are unfortunately common, and one in four people will be suffering from a mental health problem at any one time (Mental Health Foundation, 2021a). Across the NHS, we frequently use terminology that could have a wide variety of interpretations. Mental health and mental illness are perhaps two areas where this happens most commonly. As with our physical health, our mental health can be positively or negatively impacted by past experience, social factors and levels of functioning. How we function largely depends on activities of daily living, such as sleep, diet, concentration, memory, motivation and mood. It can be helpful to see mental health as a continuum, as shown in the example on page 10. It is important that our interpretation of a patient's condition does not prejudice the response, care and management that we provide to that patient and their family. This is why we need a compassionate, non-judgemental approach.

What is a mental health crisis?

A crisis can be defined by a breakdown in normal coping strategies to a nature or degree that has a significant impact on a person's mental health or functioning. A crisis is often but not always triggered by a range of adjustment challenges which can include, but are not limited to, relationship problems, finances, work pressures or bereavement. This can potentially be made worse by pre-existing history of or vulnerability to mental health conditions. How you approach the patient could mean the difference between developing a helpful therapeutic relationship and potentially heightening anxiety and escalating the severity of the situation. This is easy to imagine in a time-critical, life-threatening cardiac arrest or polytrauma patient, but when it comes to mental health it is often overlooked. The world is changing and the pressures that people face on a day-to-day basis can be the catalyst that makes someone's life unbearable, and we need to prepare for this. Often, you will be the first person who interacts with a patient in crisis, which is why it is so important to have a compassionate approach in order to facilitate de-escalation. De-escalation techniques are covered in more detail on page 27.

Parity of esteem

Parity of esteem is a concept which applies to many situations in modern society. In mental health, it has become recognised as a means for describing the inequality between physical and mental health care. Mental health patients historically do not get the same recognition as patients who present with physical health needs. This historic underinvestment has previously meant that emergency services are left bridging gaps and increasingly responding to patients in crisis. The government has sought to address this by setting out the Five Year Forward View for Mental Health (NHS England, 2016). In addition, the NHS Long Term Plan has set a commitment that the NHS will provide a single point of access to timely, universal mental health crisis care for everyone. It states that by 2024 anyone experiencing mental health crisis can call NHS 111. This is further likely to evolve to include 999, healthcare professional information and improving operational responses, with mental health ambulances staffed by ambulance clinicians and mental health crisis clinicians.

The mental health continuum

The Mental Health Continuum is a helpful guide to understanding a presenting complaint. It also provides insight on the impact of levels of functioning such as sleep, concentration, mood and memory. Like physical health, mental health is a spectrum that moves from 'excelling' to 'in crisis' dependent on a number of factors. Some considerations could include factors such as underlying conditions, vulnerability to relapse, financial status, relationships, physical health or a break from normal routine. To remain at, or move towards, the green end of the continuum

it is important to be aware of positive and negative factors that can impact our resilience. It is also helpful to think through productive and positive outlets for levels of stress and distress. For example, if we have had a hard day at work and are feeling overwhelmed, it is often more productive to talk to a trusted friend or to exercise than to turn to less productive coping strategies such as alcohol or isolation. Mental health conditions can often 'creep up' on people without them noticing. This is why it is important to objectively step back and look at where the patient is on the continuum and what positive actions or outputs can be put in place to inspire hope, recovery and moving towards the green end of the continuum.

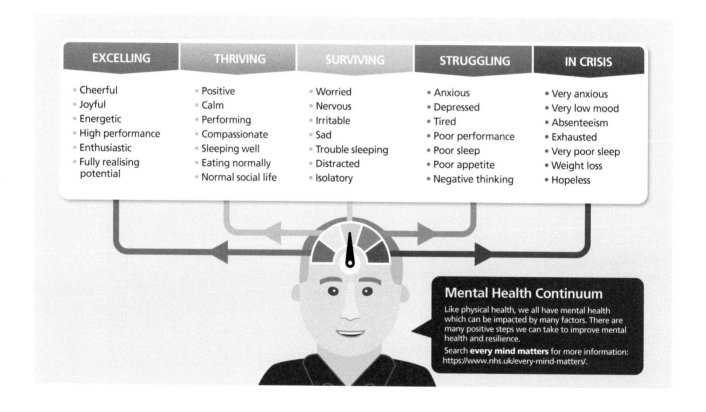

EXCELLING	THRIVING	SURVIVING	STRUGGLING	IN CRISIS
• Cheerful	• Positive	• Worried	• Anxious	• Very anxious
• Joyful	• Calm	• Nervous	• Depressed	• Very low mood
• Energetic	• Performing	• Irritable	• Tired	• Absenteeism
• High performance	• Compassionate	• Sad	• Poor performance	• Exhausted
• Enthusiastic	• Sleeping well	• Trouble sleeping	• Poor sleep	• Very poor sleep
• Fully realising potential	• Eating normally	• Distracted	• Poor appetite	• Weight loss
	• Normal social life	• Isolatory	• Negative thinking	• Hopeless

Mental Health Continuum

Like physical health, we all have mental health which can be impacted by many factors. There are many positive steps we can take to improve mental health and resilience.

Search **every mind matters** for more information: https://www.nhs.uk/every-mind-matters/.

System partnerships in the UK

Improving partnership working around mental health crisis response is a national priority. Key agencies that work together include mental health trusts, acute hospitals, ambulance service trusts, police, social services and commissioners, aiming to ensure we improve patient safety and experience. To help facilitate this national work, the Mental Health Crisis Care Concordat has been established (see: https://www.crisiscareconcordat.org.uk/). In many areas this has now developed further into integrated care systems (ICSs) or sustainability and transformation partnerships (STPs). These networks provide the opportunities to work more closely on seamless mental health care.

Crisis Care Concordat

The Crisis Care Concordat focuses on four key areas, which are:

- Recovery and staying well
- Early intervention to prevent a crisis
- Urgent/emergency care in crisis
- High-quality care to support recovery and well-being to prevent future relapse.

> A key aspect which underpins the Concordat is to ensure that 'mental health is everyone's business'.

The agreement also recognises that for too long, patients in distress have been passed between different agencies, often confusing patients and carers, along with exacerbating a crisis. The UK ambulance services, in partnership with other agencies such as NHS England and AACE, have taken the view that there is 'no wrong door' for patients presenting in crisis. Ambulance trusts, along with all healthcare providers, should be committed to supporting and enabling clinicians in ensuring that patients receive timely access to the right intervention to care and support proportionate to their needs and presentation – the first time and every time. This is increasingly being achieved with the help of key provider partners, such as mental health telephone triage within clinical contact centres for 111, 999 or healthcare professional lines, and mental health response and transport vehicles.

What does mental health and mental illness mean to you?

Across the NHS, we frequently use terminology that could have a wide variety of interpretations. Mental health and mental illness are perhaps two areas where this happens most commonly. What the general public mean when they refer to patients with a mental illness diagnosis is often different to what healthcare providers mean.

We need to be careful that our interpretation of a patient's condition does not prejudice the response, care and management that we provide to that patient and their family. This is why we need a compassionate, non-judgemental and values-based approach.

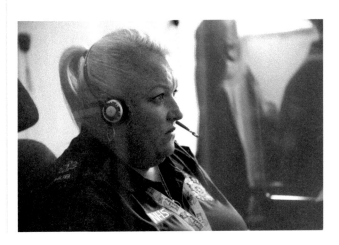

Patient quotes

When I was admitted to hospital, perhaps the only person that really seemed to care in the first few days was the paramedic who arrived in the car. She listened, held my hand and told me she'd help get me better... which at the time was what I needed. I still remember her...

Think about it, how would you like to get arrested for having a broken leg? That's what it felt like when the police took me away for being suicidal. My neighbours saw everything... I lost my dignity, my self respect and my life for nearly two years...

...They [the ambulance crew] were obviously scared that I might attack them, or do something crazy, but all I needed was them to give me time, space and to listen. Nobody listens when you have a mental illness, they all just think you're mad...

The problem is, well, when you are physically sick, people can normally tell from the way you walk or something. But when you hear voices, nobody knows but you... It's a lonely, scary place to be in, hearing things that nobody else seems to hear...

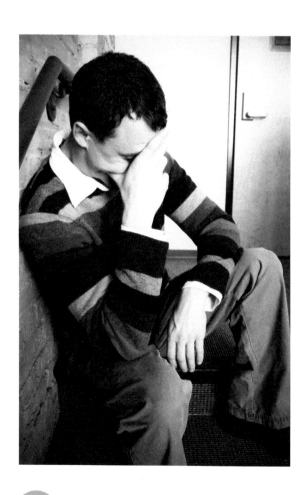

Reflective exercise

Please reflect on the following questions.

- Do you have any preconceived ideas about mental illness?

- Do you treat patients who have a mental illness differently from the way you treat patients with a physical illness?

- What feelings or emotions do you experience when treating a patient with a mental illness?

- Does society view the disability of mental illness differently from the disability associated with a physical illness?

- Do people with a mental illness expect to be treated differently by healthcare providers than those with a physical illness?

- If you or your family had a mental illness, what would you want from the ambulance crew that arrived at your door?

These are just some of the questions you might want to consider before starting to read your way through this learning material. Use the space on the next page, or a piece of paper, to jot down your thoughts and feelings. Consider how you have previously provided care to patients with a mental illness. You might want to discuss this with your crew mate, supervisor, mentor or area manager.

Activity

Personal reflections on mental health incidents

Stigma

Often we hear negative and hurtful expressions related to mental health in society, such as 'nutter', 'psycho', 'lunatic', 'waste of space'. Nearly nine out of 10 people with mental health problems say that stigma and discrimination have a negative impact on their lives (Mental Health Foundation, 2021b). We should consider some of the consequences of stigma and shame related to mental health.

Reflective exercise

Think about the consequences of stigma. Imagine if you felt lonely, hopeless, helpless, isolated and excluded and were managed as a threat. Which one of the unpleasant labels mentioned above would encourage you to access help?

Try to reflect on why we stigmatise mental health. One key reason may be that a mental health condition is unlike a physical condition, which can be difficult to see. It can also seem too complex to resolve and we do not have diagnostic equipment or easy treatment.

> '...approximately 20 out of 100 people in the UK will experience suicidal thoughts at some point during their lifetime.'
> (Mind, 2017)

Mental health: Myths and facts

Myth

Mental health problems are very rare.

Fact

The prevalence (number of people affected at any one time) of mental health problems in the UK is consistently around 25%, although this varies depending on the type of condition being examined (Mind, 2020). Anxiety and depression are amongst the most common conditions under the spectrum of mental illness. However, approximately one in five people in the UK will experience suicidal thoughts at some point during their lifetime (Mind, 2017). We consider suicide in more detail in Part 4 on pages 83–92, but you should bear in mind that it is often integrally linked with many mental health conditions (Health and Social Care Information Centre, 2009).

Myth

People with mental illness do not normally go to work.

Fact

We probably all work with someone experiencing a mental health problem. Given that one in four will be suffering at any one time, its quite likely that someone you work with is struggling with a mental health condition right now (Health and Social Care Information Centre, 2009). Why do you think they may be reticent to tell their colleagues about it?

Myth

People with mental health illnesses are usually violent and unpredictable.

Fact

People with a mental illness may be more likely to be a victim of violence.

Often, there are a number of socio-economic factors that can contribute to mental illness, such as poverty, isolation, homelessness, domestic violence, addictions and complex physical health conditions. Additionally, what is clear is that those with a mental illness are often vulnerable, and it is the vulnerable in society who experience the most violent incidents. The majority of patients experiencing mental health problems are more likely to self-harm or direct any agitation and irritability internally.

Myth

People who are weak of character, lazy or have a flawed personality are prone to a mental illness; if they corrected these personality traits, they could snap out of their illness.

Fact

Mental health problems have nothing to do with being lazy or weak. Many factors contribute to mental health problems, including:

- Biological factors, including a genetic disposition and cerebral anatomy and physiology

- Lifetime experiences, such as physical, sexual or emotional trauma

- Family history of mental health problems

- Adjustment factors such as pressures at work, in relationships or financial worries.

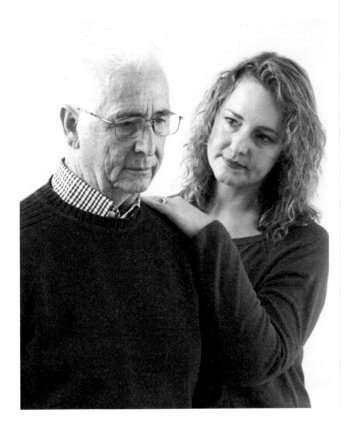

Treatment for mental illness focuses on helping the patient address each of these potential factors. We will look more closely at the causes of mental illness on pages 16–21. Bear in mind that like many medical conditions, there are a number of factors involved in developing a mental illness, just as there are a number of factors involved in developing cardiovascular disease, and in equal measure, not all of them are within the patient's direct control.

Myth

People do not recover from mental illnesses.

Fact

People can and do recover from mental illnesses. Some have a fleeting encounter with an illness, get better and never suffer from a mental illness again. Others have a relapsing or remitting pattern, where they have periods of being well, and other periods of being unwell. Part of their treatment involves helping them recognise when they are becoming unwell (relapse indicators) so that early interventions can be made before they progress further along the spectrum of illness. Have a think about how a patient's previous experiences of mental illness might influence or direct your approach to their management in the prehospital setting.

⊕ Link

For more common myths and facts about mental illness, visit the Rethink Mental Illness website:

▶ www.rethink.org

Causes of Mental Illness

In healthcare, it can sometimes be hard to frame your approach to considering why some diseases, illnesses or pathological processes affect one person and not another. It might be because of their lifestyle choices, their previous experience, their genetics, their family circumstances, a combination of these or simply due to undeterminable events. However, it is still helpful for us to understand how and why a person has been affected, not least so we can work towards removing or limiting that factor as part of their package of treatment.

Socio-economic factors

Mental health conditions are often closely linked to complex socio-economic challenges. Finances, housing, community, employment status, lifestyle, family/friend support mechanisms, drug/alcohol use and internal resilience all play key roles in mental health stability, recovery and relapse.

One way to approach any illness is to view it through the biopsychosocial model (Engel, 1977). Mental health and mental illness lend themselves particularly

well to this model. Rather than solely using the traditional biological model through which to view health and illness, the biopsychosocial model attempts to integrate other key elements which influence disease progression; it reflects how different elements can impact an individual's condition.

As illustrated in the biopsychosocial model diagram below, there are many factors which can influence why a patient might have developed a mental illness. Whilst you may sometimes think it is obvious what reasons underpin their condition, there are often multiple connected factors involved. Perhaps the complexities of these factors help explain why some conditions are so resistant to treatment in some patients.

Consider a common mental health condition, such as depression, and think more broadly about how this biopsychosocial model might begin to explain some of the contributing factors to how the condition develops in a patient. Think about some of these contributing factors as you read Karen's case study on page 20.

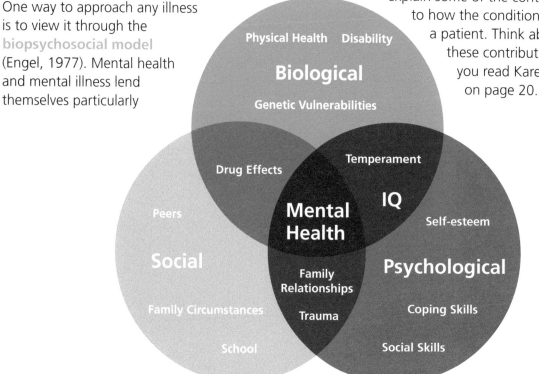

Activity

The competing factors behind mental illness

Use the activity space below and the biopsychosocial model on the previous page to classify and list examples of factors which you think might contribute to a patient developing mental illness. An example of each has been started for you.

	Factor	Example
Biological factors	Genetic susceptibility	Long family history of depression
Psychological factors	Low self-esteem	Childhood abuse
Social factors	Isolation	Single parent

BASIC STEPS tool

As of 2022, there still remains to be a validated or accredited, standardised mental health assessment tool specific to the ambulance sector to use in crisis or self-harm presentations or for those who are suicidal. The BASIC STEPS tool was developed with the intention of filling this gap, aiming to facilitate staff in completing a structured mental health and risk assessment.

The assessment tool was initially aligned to the acronym BASIC STEP (Oates, 2019), but this was updated following the pilot study. The acronym is based on several key factors, as follows (NWAS, n.d.):

Behaviour: How is the patient behaving? Is the patient engaged, withdrawn, aggressive, agitated, calm, distressed, hyperactive, hypoactive? Has their behaviour changed suddenly; what is different?

Appearance: Is the patient dressed appropriately (in relation to weather conditions, time of day, et cetera)? Is there any evidence of self-neglect? Have they self-harmed in this episode?

Speech: Is the patient speaking in a manner typical to the individual?

Insight: Does the patient acknowledge the need for help, or why you have been involved?

Cognition: Can the patient follow simple instructions? Are they orientated to date, time, place and person? Consider 4AT as required (4AT, 2021).

Set of observations: If possible, obtain observations relevant to the clinical presentation and record national early waning score (NEWS2).

Thoughts: Does the patient have thoughts of suicide, self-harm or harming others? How long have they been having these thoughts? What is the content of the thoughts and do they intend to carry them out; do they have a plan?

Emotional state: How does the patient feel, and how long have they felt like this?

Perceptual disturbances: Has the patient had any hallucinations, or do they have any delusions?

Shared decision making: What happens next for the patient? Have you considered and documented past medical history, medications and social and family history (these can be additional risk factors)? Access locally agreed pathways or personal care (safety) plans if available. Provide appropriate escalation advice and signposting, and involve or discuss with family, friends or companions if possible. Consider safeguarding, and consider the Mental Capacity Act (2005) and Mental Health Act (1983) as amended 2007 – do either apply here?

The following exceptions apply throughout: if the patient is time critical, is too violent or aggressive, declines to answer, is intoxicated or is unconscious.

⊕ Link

To find out more about the BASIC STEPS tool, see the NWAS BASIC STEPS Mental Health Assessment learning module available online:

▶ https://www.nwyhelearning.nhs.uk/elearning/northwest/NWAS/MENTAL_HEALTH/BasicSteps_2021_Update/story.html

BASIC STEPS tool

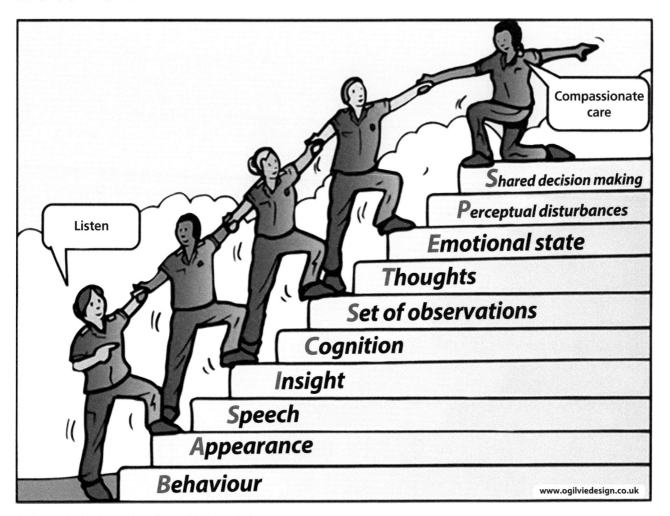

© Darren Earley. Reproduced with kind permission.

Case study – Karen

It is almost 8:30pm on your third of four night shifts in a row, and you and your colleague are called to a 18-year-old female who has taken an overdose of paracetamol. In addition, she has cut her left wrist with a razor blade, although the lacerations are believed to be superficial. Her friend called around to her address to see her, and found her lying on the sofa crying. The friend called 999 as she had no idea what to do next.

Upon arrival at the address, you see that it is a single bedsit, in a shared house for young women. The hallway is cold, the walls are dirty and upon entering Karen's room you see that she has one small living area that acts as a lounge and bedroom, with a little annexed kitchen. There is very little furniture, and although it is tidy, it looks cold, damp and unwelcoming.

Karen is sat quietly on the sofa crying, with her friend sat next to her. They tell you that she has been feeling extremely low in mood for the last six months, as her mother died last Christmas. They were very close, and they had both been physically abused by her (now estranged) father. Since her mother has died, Karen has stopped caring for herself and has often gone for several days without eating. Although she has had a few glasses of wine tonight, you feel that Karen is not intoxicated. She tells you that she often drinks quite heavily, as it 'makes the pain less real'.

You spend some time talking to Karen, and establish that she took the paracetamol five hours ago with a few glasses of wine, in the hope that she wouldn't wake up. When she did wake up, she was sad and angry that she couldn't even manage to kill herself, so she used a razor blade from a disposable razor to cut her wrist, but found the process too painful. She didn't telephone anyone, and if her friend hadn't called by she feels she would have probably tried again with the razor blade after more alcohol.

When you broach the subject of going to the hospital, Karen just shrugs her shoulders, and asks what the point is. She feels she would be better off dead right now, so there is nothing that the hospital can offer her.

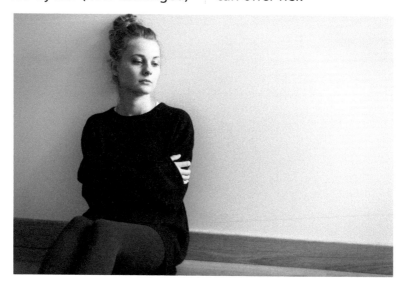

Reflective exercise

In the case study on page 20, consider the risks from a medical and mental health perspective. Think through how you might compassionately support and inspire hope for Karen, as well as who could provide professional help for her if needed.

Who do you consider accessing for additional support?

Given that Karen has expressed suicidal intent, has access to means, lives alone and has limited protective factors such as family, would you consider this a high-risk situation?

Hopefully you should be able to identify the various risk factors, and see how they each may play a part in the development of depression in the patient. If you wish, try to unpick her history, and consider how you, the GP, duty social services, an AMPH or a psychiatrist would begin to consider treating Karen. If her problems are entirely biological and potentially long term, then perhaps antidepressants are the key? However, if her problems are more social, then perhaps a referral to social services for extra assistance might be useful following initial assessment and treatment? Yet, if her background and current circumstances are interwoven, then is there a place for a combined approach of counselling, medication and social support?

Summary

In this section, we have considered how many competing interlinked factors can have an effect on the causes of mental illness, and how these might all manifest in a patient with depression. The biopsychosocial model has been explored as a framework for considering the factors which might lie behind a diagnosis of mental illness, and in the coming chapters this will act as a building block to frame your assessment of such patients, helping to underpin your risk assessment and onward referral.

⊕ Link

For another example of the biopsychosocial model and depression, see MentalHeath.net:

▶ www.mentalhelp.net

Initial Assessment of Patients with Mental Illness

The assessment process for mental illness is not particularly different to the assessment process which most paramedics and ambulance clinicians are already familiar with, and which they utilise daily for patients with physical conditions.

It is essentially a process of developing a compassionate, non-judgemental therapeutic rapport with the patient which facilitates effective communication, good listening skills and open-ended questions. This helps to gain a clear understanding of the events leading up to the current circumstances, and the ability to engage with the patient on their views of the most suitable outcome.

There is often a misconception that a mental health assessment requires the clinician to obtain a detailed understanding of the patient's mental well-being throughout their life, including their childhood, upbringing and any life events with particular emotional significance. However, on most occasions this really is not necessary in the out-of-hospital setting, and quite often gathering such detail would be distressing for the patient as well as clinically excessive. Instead, the focus should be on 'here and now circumstances', positive options and empowerment to de-escalate and manage current risks.

Longer-term treatment requires a number of interventions between the patient and their mental health clinician, at least in part because it can take this long to develop the necessary therapeutic relationship. For ambulance clinicians, it is quite acceptable to focus the assessment on current risk whilst establishing, if necessary, the most appropriate pathway going forwards in partnership with patient and carers. This needs to be sufficiently detailed so as to properly inform your clinical decisions about whether the patient needs onwards referral or signposting and, if so, where this might be most clinically appropriate.

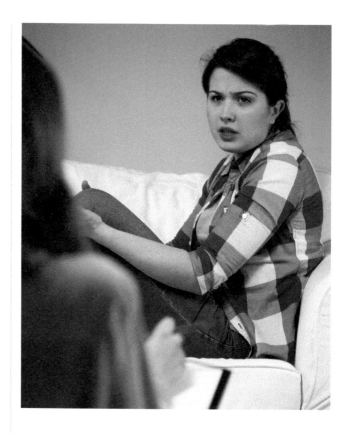

Developing a non-judgemental, compassionate rapport

As in almost all assessments, it is helpful to start with an open-ended question, which gives the patient ample opportunity to focus the conversation in the direction they feel is most beneficial. Subsequent closed questions will help the clinician more accurately focus the conversation towards the most pertinent areas of detail.

Principles of compassionate listening require a reflective non-judgemental approach that identifies concerns, inspires hope and empowers patients to explore practical, solution-focused approaches such as aspects of social prescribing described on pages 99–100.

Closed questions are those which are typically answered with either a 'yes' or 'no' response, and generally help the clinician develop a better understanding of what the patient has said by clarifying finer detail. If closed questions are used too much or too soon, they can impact the flow of conversation and give the patient an impression that the clinician does not want them to expand on or explore their story.

Open questions are those that cannot easily be answered by a simple 'yes' or 'no' answer. These types of questions broaden the area of conversation between the clinician and the patient, and give the patient permission to explore their emotions and the areas of concern most important to them at that time. If at all possible, try not to interrupt the initial response from the patient, as the uninterrupted flow helps build an initial rapport.

It is really important to develop a therapeutic rapport. Compassion, warmth, empathy and full attention can help de-escalate any distress or escalating situations. Focus on a low-stimulus environment where you can discuss the situation. Where possible and appropriate with the patient, remove or distract any emotive or distressed audience, or excessive stimulus and distraction such as loud music or television. Include choices and outcomes and empower the patient to make informed decisions around what would help right now.

Clinical tip

Next time you assess a patient, try opening the consultation with a broad, open question, such as:

'Can you tell me what has happened today?'

Even when you do not interrupt, patients often may not speak for much more than 30 seconds but they will feel that they have been given the chance to explain their concerns without distraction.

During the initial assessment, try and get a good, clear understanding of what the patient's current concerns are. Be clear in your head what the priority is for the patient, and whether that seems consistent with how they are presenting non-verbally. Subsequently, closed questions can be used to get a better understanding of other key elements, including: previous medical and psychiatric history; previous involvement with mental health services; current prescribed medications and degree of concordance; social circumstances, including current employment and relationship status; drug and alcohol use, both currently and in the past; and any forensic or criminal background (where necessary).

We may not have all the answers but by compassionately working together with the patients we can inspire hope and trust and reduce distress.

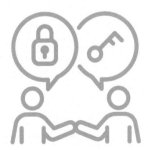

The mental state assessment

Once you have a firm understanding of the patient's story, current problems and relevant previous history, you should move on to performing a brief mental health assessment. In much the same way as a physical assessment of a medical patient involves auscultating the chest, palpating the abdomen or testing sensation, the mental state assessment is a structured way of considering pertinent elements of the patient's current mental state. It involves observation of how the patient interacts with others, combined with focused questions about specific psychiatric symptoms. It also involves non-verbal presentation such as posture, engagement, facial expressions, emotions and communication elements such as pitch, tone and volume.

Managing agitation and distress in patients with a mental illness

Perhaps one of the most perturbing scenarios for all community clinicians is an agitated and distressed patient. Please remember, there is no reason to suggest that this behaviour is any more likely to be encountered in patients with a mental illness than in patients with a physical ailment. Nonetheless, scenarios do occur where the clinician is required to try and assess and manage an agitated or distressed patient, and there are a number of approaches that may be used.

There may be situations where the patient is far too agitated for safe approach, and in no way should clinicians place themselves at risk of injury from any agitated patient presenting with either a physical or a mental health condition. If they require assessment or treatment and you deem it unsafe to approach, then follow local policy for requesting police or security assistance where clinically indicated (Davies and Craig, 1998).

However, in many cases, potentially distressing scenarios can be managed and contained by the clinicians involved and, just like many other areas of medicine, de-escalation skills, scene safety and dynamic risk assessment are strengths in themselves. It takes time, practice and effort to become confident and capable at communicating with distressed patients, but generally ambulance staff tend to have both aptitude and experience with this (Davies and Craig, 1998).

Clinical tip

The reasons that patients become agitated are often underpinned by fear, frustration and a sense of losing control. Most adults develop a typical coping strategy to deal with stress-provoking situations, and in general these are well adapted for normal stressful events. However, some patients have less effective coping strategies. Others have a low threshold for their usual strategies and become overwhelmed when stressed. In both these scenarios, the patient's behaviour can quickly become agitated. Part of your job is to help put them back in control, de-escalate, inspire hope, provide realistic solution-focused options or reassure them that you are there to help.

Recognising distress

Most clinicians in the prehospital setting can quickly recognise distress, but the important thing is not to respond to the distress in a way that exacerbates it. In the early stages, this distress might be directed at you, as the clinician, but you should not take this personally. Remaining calm and relaxed will help prevent unnecessary escalation.

Reflecting distress

Reflecting distress can demonstrate that you empathise with the patient, and are prepared to co-operate with them to help find a solution. You should reflect back their highly expressed emotions in a more balanced and less emotional manner. Perhaps in response to the statement 'you do not care, you do not want to help me', you might reflect back the statement 'I am sorry that you feel that way' and 'what can we do now to help improve the current situation?'.

Modelling appropriate behaviour (behaviour breeds behaviour)

When we demonstrate courtesy, dignity and respect we are more likely to receive the same values back. During any conversation, people often begin to mirror each others' individual terms, gestures or actions, which helps form meaningful connection and understanding (Iacoboni, 2008). By remaining calm, focused and engaged, you can demonstrate to the patient that this is the type of behaviour that you would like to observe from them too. Escalating your tone or using confrontational body language can sometimes mirror the same outcomes back at you.

Identifying goals

It is best to identify goals in a co-operative and mutually agreeable manner, whilst ensuring that your therapeutic aims are involved in the plan. It might be that you feel the patient needs a referral to a particular service, but you need to negotiate how and when they attend this meeting so that they feel empowered by and included in the decisions. Obviously, the severity of their illness might very much dictate the degree of agreement or their capacity to consent which can be obtained.

Key reflections

Try to imagine being in the patient's shoes. They may be in pain, anxious, have faced a long delay, have had previous bad experiences, be overwhelmed by many factors, be influenced by an audience or distressed relative or feel hopeless, helpless or that nobody cares. Distress and anger are short-lived emotions. Acknowledging the distress and engaging in a calm and compassionate way provides positive choices and outcomes, giving you the best opportunity to de-escalate an escalating situation. Having a non-judgemental approach and listening attentively to concerns helps the patient realise their concerns may be valid and justified.

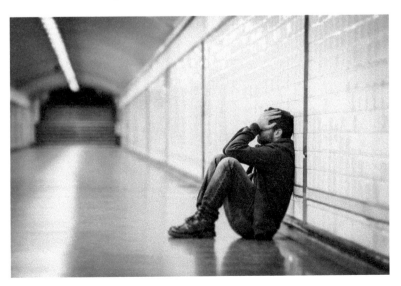

Clinical tip

You might find that using this approach to reflect on distress triggers is also helpful in many other situations unrelated to mental health where parties become agitated, distressed or potentially confrontational, including family disagreements, work conflicts or simply when negotiating with friends! For example, we can all feel irritable and irrational when our resilience is tested. A scenario where we may be tired, stressed, overwhelmed or worried might affect our objectivity. A good example is that of road rage, which we often see where people beep horns and make angry gestures when in traffic congestion.

Link

For an example of how mental health can affect all of us, see the video under the link below.

Transport for London: Share the Road, M&C Saatchi London

▶ www.youtube.com/watch?v=ObTkJpVJgs8

Dynamic Risk Assessment and Management Plans

There are two key aspects to consider when safely assessing and managing risk. These are probability and severity.

When considering **probability**, we look at how likely is it that the situation will occur. When considering **severity**, we look at the potential level of impact of the risk. We know we apply proportionate, positive risk-taking behaviour all the time. An obvious example is driving a car. To reduce the probability of an accident occurring, we ensure the car is in a good state of repair, serviced with an up-to-date MOT. We would also ensure we are not too tired or impaired in any way to drive. We mitigate the severity of a potential accident by wearing a seatbelt and having airbags and other safety factors in our car. Considering this example, it is important to note that we do take positive, proportionate risks all the time and we need to consider all factors in managing risks.

 Risk is a **fluid and dynamic process** that changes all the time.

Reflective exercise

Try to reflect on the risk management chart below and consider some scenarios where you responded to incidents and safely considered all the risk factors to achieve a positive outcome.

Dynamic risk management

Examples of risk

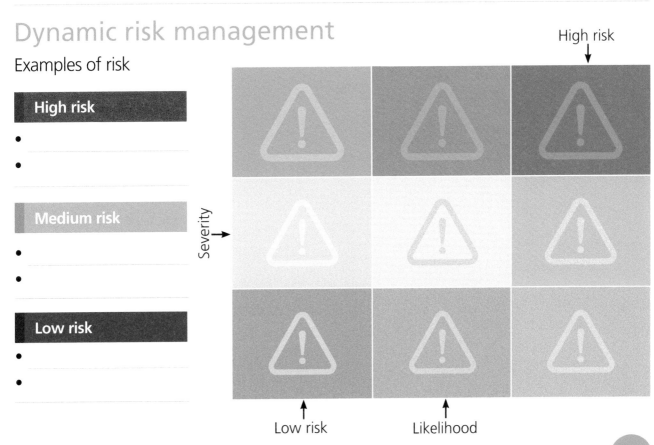

The eight 'S' principles

Awareness of, understanding and proportionately managing risk is a priority in keeping staff and patients safe. To minimise risk we need to constantly evaluate safety considering a number of factors, bearing in mind that risk is fluid and situations can change. From the beginning of calls through to control rooms we need to consider all possible risk factors, continually applying the eight 'S' principles as outlined below.

S THE EIGHT 'S' PRINCIPLES

02 Scene safety

Before entering, is the scene unsafe in any way? Are there relatives, friends or neighbours that may be a risk? Are there dangerous dogs or other animals? Is the environment unsafe in any way? How is the patient presenting? Are they calm and co-operative or anxious and distressed? Are they agitated, threatening or raising their voice? If you have some concerns about levels of distress, always consider an exit route and minimise obstacles or people within that exit route. Utilise your employer's escalation process with radio support and reflect back on your conflict resolution training.

03 Speech

Is the patient raising their voice or using unhelpful language? Can you reduce levels of noise or audiences if exacerbating the situation? Consider your speech, pitch, tone and volume. Avoid using jargon which patients will not understand. Communicate with compassion, warmth, empathy and a non-judgemental approach. Imagine what it would be like being in their shoes or having a loved one with a similar condition or presentation. Be personable in order to connect with the patient in distress; for example, showing (where appropriate) the same interests, such as football team, family interests or local community interests.

01 Situational awareness

En route to the incident think about the nature of the call, any precipitating factors, any known previous risks and any warning markers that would require additional support.

05 Stance

Consider how you hold and move your body. An open posture with good eye contact, without folded arms or hands in pockets, provides a helpful framework to reassure and de-escalate.

04 Space

Typically, we tolerate space with close friends and trusted colleagues at roughly the distance of an arm's length. If a patient is anxious or distressed it may be appropriate (where possible) to at least double this distance, whilst considering the need to communicate and build a therapeutic rapport.

06 Stability

If a patient is agitated, consider a slightly side-on approach with legs roughly shoulder-width apart. This stance is less confrontational, and you are a smaller target so it is easier to defend yourself.

08 Safeguarding

If a patient presents as an ongoing risk of vulnerability, neglect or a risk to someone else, always remember to consult other relevant professionals in the decision-making and pathways process and remember to safeguard if concerns are raised using your employer's processes.

07 Support following

Where possible, think about re-establishing a rapport, particularly if there was only a minor level of anxiety or agitation. At some point we need to negotiate a positive outcome even with the assistance of other professionals such as social workers, mental health professionals, security or police. Remember, although we do face some challenging situations patients can be both distressed and vulnerable, particularly within a life-threatening scenario. If helpful, think about a debrief or support with your crewmate or line manager.

Influential factors

Here are some example (patient and environment) factors that could influence anxiety and agitation in either a medical or mental health incident (this list is not exhaustive).

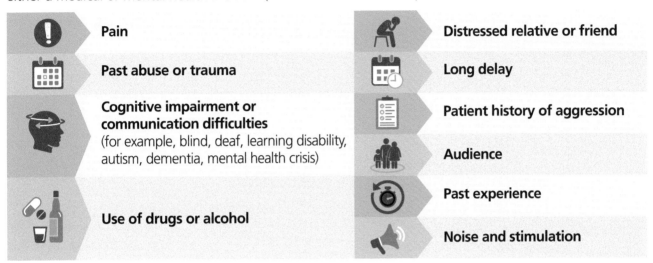

Pain	**Distressed relative or friend**
Past abuse or trauma	**Long delay**
Cognitive impairment or communication difficulties (for example, blind, deaf, learning disability, autism, dementia, mental health crisis)	**Patient history of aggression**
	Audience
	Past experience
Use of drugs or alcohol	**Noise and stimulation**

Staff factors

There is only one staff factor that can either positively or negatively impact an outcome or incident: your approach. Please see pages 93–104 for more information on employee mental health and resilience.

Reflective exercise

- Is it not **human to have our resilience tested** at times?
- Think about **rational objectivity**.
- **What factors may impact your resilience**? (For example, back-to-back incidents, confidence in dealing with a particular type of incident, past experience, personal challenges.)
- Have you ever worked with **a colleague who has contributed to escalating levels of distress**?
- Have you ever **done or said something in the heat of the moment which you later regretted**?

- If you feel a situation is impacting your level of anxiety or irritability, would it help to take time to **stop and think**, where possible?
- Could it be **best to ask a colleague to take over**?
- **Could the patient feel more comfortable with a colleague of the same sex**?
- What are the best possible ways to reach a positive outcome when considering **role, boundaries, human factors, empowerment, negotiation and limit setting**?

Keys to limit setting

☑ Establish **clear boundaries**	☑ **Be calm, rational** and **objective**	☑ **Always act in the patient's best interests,** with any intervention being reasonable and proportionate to the presenting situation and any direct intervention being the least restrictive option.
☑ Explain what is **within your gift** to support	☑ Explain clearly a **particular course of action** and **why it is necessary**	
☑ Make every effort to **co-produce best outcome with patient** and any available supportive relatives or friends	☑ **Be clear on consequences** if patient refuses and consider capacity	
☑ Think about the **'ask first, then tell, then act' approach**		

Case study – Rashid

You are called to Rashid, a 22-year-old man, by his best friend, as she has become increasingly concerned for his well-being. Upon arrival at a university-owned campus tower block you are met by Rashid's friend at the front door; she tells you that their flat is on the ninth floor and she will show you the way. Whilst riding in the elevator, she begins to recite the recent events to you.

Rashid is, according to his friend, a very clever guy. He finished college

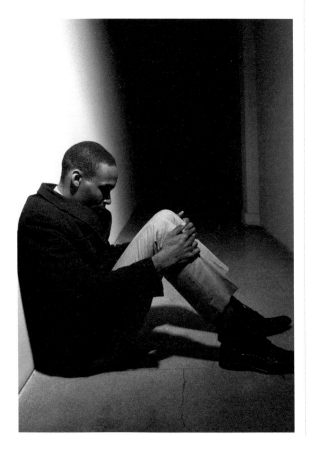

with great A-level results, and is doing a marketing course at university. He is in his second year now, and has a large group of friends that he made on the course during his first year. Since the start of the second year, he has been much more withdrawn. At first, everyone thought this was because his mother was unwell and he was worried about her. He has started to skip lectures, and rarely attends social events any more. On the odd occasion that he has gone out, he has left early, after appearing uncomfortable in the presence of a large group.

Over the weekend, he has spent almost every minute in his room. There has been some unusual shouting, but his friends thought this was an argument Rashid was having over the phone with his brother. Tonight, however, Rashid has been pacing the corridor outside of his room. He refuses to go back inside his room as he says it has been remotely bugged by the CIA.

Upon entering the flat, it appears tidy and clean. Rashid is sat on the floor at the end of the corridor, wearing jeans and a blazer. When you speak to him, he answers quietly and in short sentences. He appears distracted, sometimes looking up to the left as if responding to something or somebody. He doesn't give much away about how he is feeling, but he does admit that he is frightened.

Activity

Planning your assessment

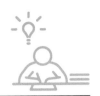

Clearly Rashid is unwell, and needs further assessment. However, there are no time-critical, medical features to his condition, and therefore it is appropriate to spend some time with him, getting a better understanding of what he is experiencing and developing an early therapeutic relationship.

1. What questions are you going to ask Rashid in the next 10 minutes? Is there anything in particular that you think would be particularly important?

2. Using the blank assessment tool below, begin to fill out your impression of Rashid's condition. Whilst you may not know all the information at this point, jot down what you think you might find out with more appropriate questions to ask or cross reference. Think about views of family, friends or healthcare professionals where available and appropriate from a confidentiality, risk and consent perspective.

3. Think about how you will structure your telephone referral to the crisis team or other referral agency.

4. What options are available to you if Rashid does not want to attend hospital and you feel he is a high risk to himself or others?

(The Mental Health Act and issues of capacity will be covered in the 'Legal Framework and Decision Making' section on pages 34–44.)

Appearance

Thoughts

Speech

Perception

Mood and affect

Orientation

Case study – Mae

You are called to a new housing estate on the edge of the local town. While you have never been here before, you are aware that the properties are reputed to be large and expensive!

The call is to a 60-year-old female called Mae. The call has been placed by a local GP, who wants assistance in transferring Mae to the local mental health unit. Upon arrival, the GP and the social worker are outside the house, and there are a number of police vehicles in the street.

The GP tells you that Mae has no prior history of mental health problems. Given the current presentation, a Mental Health Act assessment has been carried out and Mae has been detained under Section 2 of the Mental Health Act. This means she will be taken to a mental health hospital for assessment and treatment due to being a risk to herself as well as others. She is retired from her role as a school teacher, and lives with her husband in the property. Mae's husband has made the call this evening, as he has found Mae to become increasingly chaotic as the day has progressed. She awoke early yesterday morning, and has hardly slept since. She has cleaned the house from top to bottom, and spent much of the evening in the garden, hoovering the grass and tending to her plants. When he asked her to come inside, Mae shouted at her husband, and carried on, despite it being nearly 11:00pm in the winter.

Once Mae eventually came inside, she has been agitated, ranting and raving at her husband in an almost incoherent manner. She has shown him a number of recent bank statements that show very excessive spending over the last few weeks on irrational items, and he suspects the total may be in the thousands of pounds.

You approach Mae in an attempt to introduce yourself and gauge whether she will be safe to travel with you in the ambulance, unaccompanied by the police. You notice that she is wearing an unusual combination of clothing, including a large sun hat and bright green trousers. Unfortunately, she screams and shouts at you in an almost incoherent manner, and threatens to attack you, confirming your suspicion that she will need to be transported with the police in attendance.

En route to hospital, Mae is much less aggressive, but continues to rant. Her train of thought appears to be very muddled, and you struggle to follow her conversation. She seems to change from angry and offended to laughing and jovial within a matter of minutes.

Activity
Thinking about the differentials

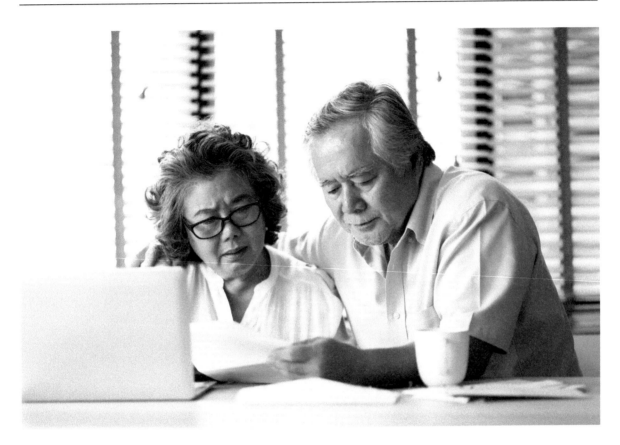

1. Mae is demonstrating a number of signs and symptoms typical of more than one mental health condition. On the face of the information provided, what are your top two differential diagnoses for Mae?

2. Are there any medical conditions that you can think of that might lead to someone acting in such a manner?

3. If you were to plan Mae's care in the hospital for the next 24 hours, what considerations would you make? (Do not worry about making a formal management plan, but think more broadly about what issues the doctors and mental health nurses might need to cover.)

Think about Mae's:

- Safety

- Dignity

- Human rights

- Mental well-being

- Physical well-being.

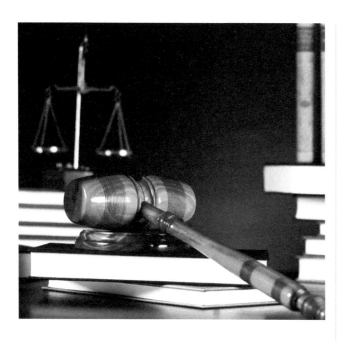

The main aspects of legislation relevant to the ambulance service and incidents involving patients with mental health conditions are the Mental Health Act (MHA), Mental Capacity Act (MCA) and the Liberty Protection Safeguards (LPS) which will replace the Deprivation of Liberty Safeguards (DoLS) system (Department of Health & Social Care, 2021). These encompass concepts around Best Interests decision making, compassionate care, empowerment, safety, proportionality and duty of care.

The Mental Health Act

The MHA covers the compulsory admission to hospital and detention within hospital of patients experiencing severe mental health problems that require either assessment or treatment.

Patients can only be detained under the MHA by an approved mental health professional (AMHP) and two appropriately qualified doctors. The main sections relevant to the ambulance service are Section 2, Section 3 and Sections 135 (1), 135 (2) and 136 (police holding powers). Patients

already on leave whilst on a Section 2 or 3 can be compulsorily brought back to hospital if their mental state deteriorates whilst on leave.

Section 136 relates to the police's ability to compulsorily detain and take a patient to a 'place of safety' in order to be assessed under the MHA. Section magistrates' court warrant 135 (1) is the same as 136 except that it relates to entering and detaining a patient in their own home as opposed to in a community setting. The police require a court magistrate's warrant (applied for by an AMHP) and an AMHP to action a Section 135 (1).

Patients can only be detained under the MHA or taken to a place of safety for assessment where there is a high threshold of risk. These include where there is an identified or suspected mental illness, where there is evidence of a significant and current risk of harm to self or others or where there is a risk of severe neglect or possible further significant deterioration in their illness. All reasonable efforts should be made to explore alternative options to compulsory detention, and, where clinically indicated, voluntary or 'informal admission' should be considered.

Transporting patients under the Act

Your involvement when a patient is detained is likely to be as a means of safe, compassionate conveyance of a patient who is being admitted under the section. They are a healthcare patient, rather than a custodial candidate, and therefore, if safe, it is always preferable that they are transported by ambulance; this can also help negate perceived stigma within the community, as outlined in the revised MHA Code of Practice (Department of Health, 2015). In rare occasions where there is an active risk of aggression or abscondence, a dynamic risk assessment between the AMHP and/or police should be undertaken. In some circumstances, it may be helpful for both the

Mental Health Act (MHA)

2

Section 2 – Applied for by an AMHP with medical recommendations from two doctors, or (very rarely) by nearest relative. The patient can be detained and admitted for up to 28 days for assessment under the authority of two doctors.

3

Section 3 – Applied for by an AMHP or the nearest relative where a diagnosis is already known. Allows up to six months of treatment under the authority of two doctors, one of whom is Section 12 approved.

4

Section 4 – An emergency 72-hour admission under the authority of one Section 12 doctor, or a GP who has seen the patient in the past 24 hours. Applied for by an AMHP or the nearest relative.

5(2)

Section 5(2) – A holding power exercised by doctors on a ward to detain informally admitted patients for up to 72 hours.

5(4)

Section 5(4) – An emergency holding power exercised by a mental health or learning disability nurse on a hospital ward to detain informally admitted patients for up to six hours.

6

Section 6 – 'An application for the admission of a patient to a hospital shall be sufficient authority for the applicant, or any person authorised by the applicant, to take the patient and convey him to the hospital.' This provides ambulance services with authority to convey.

17

Section 17 – Leave is given to patients as part of their recovery and rehabilitation. Leave can be brief initially but then built up to extended periods of time. If a patient does not return when they have been granted leave, they are considered absent without leave (AWOL).

135(1)

Section 135(1) – A power granted by a magistrate at the request of an AMHP to allow police accompanied by an AMHP to:

- Gain entry to private premises due to levels of mental health concerns where patient is refusing entry.

This also grants the power to:

- Remove the patient to a place of safety (POS) for assessment to be conducted (could include own home as a POS)

- A warrant may be progressed even if access can be obtained.

135(2)

Section 135(2) – Allows a constable or another person authorised under the MHA to apply for a warrant to gain entry to premises, and retake and return an AWOL patient (for example, Section 17 leave). It also covers community treatment orders (CTOs) where the detained patient has not attended when recalled to hospital. A power of detention for AWOL patients exists under Section 18 MHA which also carries a power of arrest. Section 18 itself does not have a power of entry. The warrant is required when entry to the premises is or will be refused.

136

Section 136 – A power to allow police officers to remove a person from a public place (not a home or private garden or outbuilding) for a mental health assessment at a health-based POS where there is a need for immediate care or control. Police should liaise with key clinicians to support decision making prior to detention where practically possible.

police and the ambulance service to be involved in the conveyance, in order to manage the mental health, safety and security of the admission. The AMHP will be a useful source of reference in deciding the least restrictive, most therapeutic form of transport (this is outlined in detail within the updated Mental Health Act 1983: Code of Practice (Department of Health, 2015)). Patients being transferred from a public or private mental health hospital should ideally have an escort, not necessarily an AMHP, along with an Authority to Convey form and Section papers.

In the case of Section 136, patients should be transported by an ambulance on the principle that a health-based condition should have a health-based response. The police should accompany the clinician and the patient either in the vehicle or following behind, based on presenting risk assessment. However, if the patient is travelling in the police vehicle due to high risk of aggression or absconding, then the most senior ambulance clinician should travel in the police vehicle with the ambulance following behind.

For transfers between mental health facilities, there should be an escort from the ward. If the patient has been sedated, an escort must be present. Where clinically indicated, a mental health nurse escort should be provided. Section papers and Authority to Convey forms should also be present.

Summary

The threshold for compulsory detention under the MHA is high.

It is used where there is evidence of a significant risk to the patient or to others. If the patient presents in mental health crisis and refuses treatment or conveyance, assess and document the risks and escalation process. Remember, the MHA is for mental health risks. For example, refer to Sessay vs SLAM: the case conclusion was that the MHA should have been utilised instead of the MCA as there was not an immediate, life-saving medical need and the MHA supersedes the MCA in these scenarios (R (Sessay) v South London and Maudsley NHS Foundation Trust, 2011). If the patient presents with an immediate, serious or life-threatening medical

condition then the MCA is a more appropriate process. A frequent example would be toxic overdose with alcohol, which would require medical treatment under the MCA prior to MHA assessment. We will move on to the MCA in the next section.

Reflective exercise

Try to imagine you or one of your loved ones being 'in the shoes' of the detained patient. They may already feel anxiety, shame and distress about being admitted against their will. Mental illness is a health-based condition and a detained patient has not committed any crime. This is why it is important to have wherever possible a compassionate health-based transport solution.

Mental Capacity Act 2005

The MCA is an Act of Parliament intended to protect those who may lack the capacity to make decisions about their care (Department for Constitutional Affairs, 2007). The first principle of the MCA is that a person must be assumed to have capacity to make a decision or act for themselves unless it is established that they lack capacity in relation to those matters. It is important to note that an unwise decision does not imply a lack of capacity.

In order to assess capacity, patients need to be able to understand the treatment options open, the potential risks and feedback on this information. Typically, there are a range of areas where patients may lack capacity to consent to treatment. There may for example be a number of physical health problems such as head injury, UTI, hypoxia, hypoglycaemia, alcohol or drug intoxication or cognitive impairments. Cognitive impairments can sometimes include dementia, learning disabilities and severe mental illness, although this list is not exhaustive. Patients can also be temporarily impaired from informed decision making and examples of this include patients who are severely intoxicated or under the influence of drugs.

Where there is evidence of impaired capacity, clinicians need to make a best interests decision on treatment or conveyance. It is important to note that clinicians need to demonstrate they have taken reasonable steps to negotiate on options and best interests. Any persuasion or physical intervention (restraint) must be proportionate to the likelihood and potential severity of harm. Appropriate risk assessment and management on available resources must be considered. This should be from the perspective of the clinician's personal safety and the level of urgency or severity of risk to the patient's condition.

When to consider using the Act

You should assume that a patient has capacity unless they give you reason to doubt it. See the five MCA principles on page 38.

Where patients are intoxicated through drink or drugs, or are suffering from severe emotional distress, you must be satisfied that these temporary factors are operating to such a degree that they lack capacity. Often this will be due to the patient's inability to weigh up information

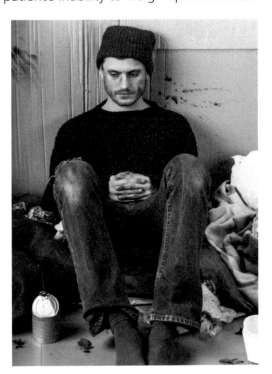

You may have concerns due to:

- The patient's behaviour
- The patient's circumstances
- Concerns raised by someone else
- Knowledge of a long-term condition such as dementia
- Failed or threatened suicide attempts
- Possible drug or alcohol intoxication.

Please note that an unwise decision does not necessarily indicate lack of capacity.

(see stage two (third question) of the mental capacity assessment tool on page 38).

If a patient lacks capacity, Section 5 and Section 6 of the MCA highlight all reasonable steps which are in the person's best interests to be taken to prolong their life. The MCA only applies to individuals aged 16 years and above.

The three-stage mental capacity assessment

The MCA covers medical presentations and risks related to informed decision making. Where a patient refuses treatment, the three-stage functional test must be completed and clearly documented. Examples of situations where patients could lack capacity include (but are not limited to): hypoglycaemia, concussion, intoxication, head injury, mental health crisis, infection or dementia. There are **five key principles** which underpin the MCA 2005.

In assessing whether a person can make their own decision or lacks the mental capacity at the time, three key issues should be considered: can the person make the decision at the time it needs to be made? Do they have a disturbance in the functioning of the mind or brain? Is it this disturbance to is preventing the person being able to make the decision?

The causative nexus is the link between a person's disturbance of functioning and their ability to make a particular decision at the time it needs to be made. For example, someone with a history of depression may struggle less with decision making when they

The five MCA principles

1	2	3	4	5
A person must be assumed to have capacity, unless it is established that they lack capacity. (Complete the three-stage mental capacity assessment if consent refused or cannot consent and risk of serious harm.)	A person is not to be treated as unable to make a decision unless all practical steps to help them do so have been taken without success.	A person is not to be treated as unable to make a decision merely because they make an unwise decision.	An act or decision made for a person who lacks capacity must be done in their best interests.	Before the act is done, or the decision is made, you must consider whether the outcome can be achieved in a way that is less restrictive.

The three-stage mental capacity assessment tool

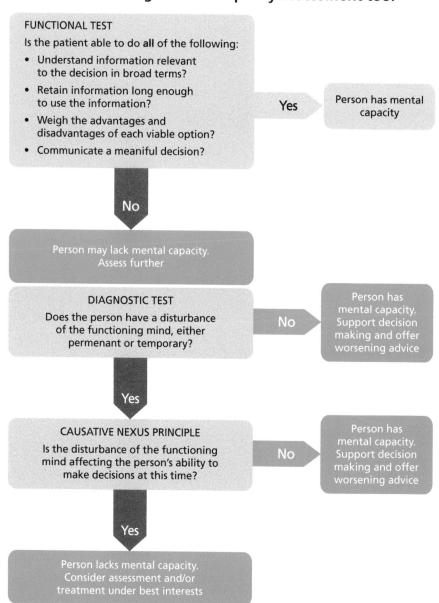

FUNCTIONAL TEST
Is the patient able to do **all** of the following:
- Understand information relevant to the decision in broad terms?
- Retain information long enough to use the information?
- Weigh the advantages and disadvantages of each viable option?
- Communicate a meaniful decision?

Yes → Person has mental capacity

No ↓

Person may lack mental capacity. Assess further

DIAGNOSTIC TEST
Does the person have a disturbance of the functioning mind, either permenant or temporary?

No → Person has mental capacity. Support decision making and offer worsening advice

Yes ↓

CAUSATIVE NEXUS PRINCIPLE
Is the disturbance of the functioning mind affecting the person's ability to make decisions at this time?

No → Person has mental capacity. Support decision making and offer worsening advice

Yes ↓

Person lacks mental capacity. Consider assessment and/or treatment under best interests

Assessing Capacity in an Emergency Situation

Does this patient want to make a decision about their care that you consider unwise, refusing either treatment or transport to hospital?

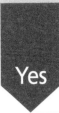 **No** → Treat to normal protocols and JRCALC and Trust guidelines.

Yes ↓

Is the patient under 16 years of age?

Yes → Where possible, gain parental consent if the patient is under 16.

Gillick Competence
A child can consent if they have sufficient understanding and intelligence to fully understand what is involved in a proposed treatment. However, their refusal to consent to emergency treatment can be overridden by a person with parental responsibility.

For Patients of All Ages
Make best-interests decision.

Use persuasion and try to prevent further harm.

Consider assistance and support from family, police, social care, CAMHS, Mental Health Team or GP, OOH, CSD team.

No ↓

Decide if the patient is competent to refuse treatment or transport by completing the three-stage mental capacity assessment for each decision required. Does the patient have capacity to make this decision?

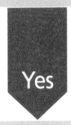 **No** → **Document thoroughly** full details of three-stage mental capacity assessment.

Consider patient's past and present wishes and feelings, such as an advance directive to refuse treatment.

Consider the beliefs and values that are likely to influence a decision should they have capacity, such as a Jehovah's witness refusing a blood transfusion.

Yes ↓

Ensure **documentation** is completed as per normal protocols.

Ensure involvement with local mental health service/crisis team, family (where possible and appropriate) and any other relevant professionals to support decision making.

If patient is not transported, then where possible arrange for them to be with a responsible adult and document who this is.

Ensure thorough safety netting, providing advice to both patient and carer/family if not proportionate to intervene or convey.

Explain to patient and carers to call again should the patient reconsider their decision.

Where possible, ensure onward referral, with consent, to GP or others as appropriate.

Where a patient is in immediate risk, the ability to undertake a full and thorough assessment of their mental capacity is not always possible (for example, a patient with reduced consciousness or catastrophic haemorrhage). In such circumstances, decisions must be made based on the evidence available at that time and on the principle that the balance of probabilities (that is, being more likely than not) would suggest that the patient lacked capacity. The principles around urgent and life-saving treatment are covered under S5 and S6 of the MCA.

Any actions then undertaken on this basis must be considered immediately necessary to save life and and/or prevent serious deterioration in the patient's physical or mental well-being.
This doctrine is a positive duty in law, which means that failure to act could be deemed negligent.

are not acutely depressed. However, depression can cause a person to think in very concrete terms and impact on a person's ability to think in more abstract terms (for example, how their life could be better at some stage in the future). This could mean a suicidal patient who appears able to answer questions and retain information may still lack the mental capacity to consent to treatment as they are unable to accurately weigh relevant information, especially if they are experiencing emotional dysregulation at the time. To give another example, a person with dementia may not be able to retain new information relevant to the decision they need to make due to the impact some forms of dementia can have on memory and other executive functioning skills.

Reasonable force

There is no legal definition of reasonable force; however, in practical terms it is the minimum amount of force required to achieve the desired outcome, and it will change dependent on the situation to protect yourself and, in the context of the MCA, to treat a patient.

For example, the amount of force required to defend life might be greater than that to defend property. Ambulance staff not currently trained in safe holding should only forcibly hold a patient as a last resort in an emergency and it should be to preserve life in balance with the personal safety of ambulance staff.

Clinical tip

Remember, the clinician making a decision on someone else's behalf needs to be able to justify that decision and the steps taken must be proportionate and well documented. Where possible, carers should be consulted but the ultimate decision on capacity lies with the clinician.

Removing under MCA (Section 5 and Section 6)	Liberty Protection Safeguards (LPS) (formerly DoLS)
These sections allow for patients to be restrained and escorted to hospital for any emergency or urgent treatment considerations if the patient lacks capacity.	While LPS only applies to hospital and care home settings, ambulance and police staff may with further assessment be asked to return a patient subject to LPS to a care home or hospital.
This must be in the patient's best interests and proportionate to the likelihood and seriousness of the risk of harm to the patient. Removal is in response to the risk of greater harm to the patient if they are not removed. Any physical intervention has to be a last resort and proportionate to the risk. Please ensure it is documented and escalated robustly.	The police and ambulance service cannot use LPS as it applies to the authorised location only, however the MCA or MHA could be used to transport a patient in an emergency if it is in their best interests.

Further reading

Eaton, G. 2019. *Law and Ethics for Paramedics: An Essential Guide* (1st Edn). Bridgwater: Class Professional Publishing.

Case studies

Utilise your conflict resolution skills and remember to consult patients, family and friends where possible. Escalate and access help if needed through line management, a clinical contact centre (CCC), a clinical support desk (CSD), mental health nurses, partners such as crisis teams, street triage, on-call AMHPs, GPs or the police and mental health triage hubs. Please **clearly** document your decision-making process, particularly on complex incidents.

Dave

Dave is a 35-year-old male with a history of diabetes.

You are called to Dave who is having a 'hypo'. Dave is confused and irritable but not aggressive or combative. You quickly determine that Dave lacks capacity after completing the two-stage test and make a best interest decision to treat him. The decision is made on the basis that as a clinician you have a positive duty to preserve life. You do a BM test and treat with glucose via the most suitable clinical means and the least amount of physical safe-holding. Upon Dave's recovery, you use a compassionate approach to inform him of your decision-making process and document your mental capacity assessment and clinical intervention.

Doris

Doris is an 85-year-old female living alone with confusion and early onset dementia.

You suspect Doris is in a state of neglect and has a query UTI. She is confused and as a clinician on scene you determine that she lacks capacity, following consideration of her views and calls to any available family or friends. You consider an assessment of the risk to Doris for further deterioration and risk to yourself from carrying out physical intervention. You determine that the 'least restrictive, last resort and reasonable and proportionate' action would be to gently guide Doris with low-level arm immobilisation to a place or position of assessment and or treatment. You then document your decision-making process, including thorough completion of the MCA decision-making process and safeguarding referral for neglect.

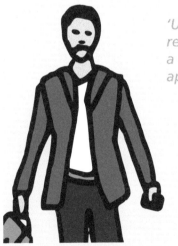

'Upon Dave's recovery, you use a compassionate approach...'

'...gently guide Doris with low-level arm immobilisation to a place or position of assessment and or treatment.'

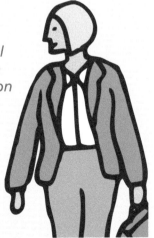

Case studies (continued)

Sameera

Sameera is a 22-year-old female with a history of depression.

Sameera has been assessed under the MHA by an AMHP and two suitably trained doctors. She is detained under Section 2. You have been asked to convey Sameera to hospital and are provided with the detention papers and conveyance forms. On arrival at the hospital Sameera becomes restless, anxious and distressed. You determine that as she is detained under the MHA you should do all you can to persuade, de-escalate and prevent Sameera from absconding. After compassionate de-escalation and low-level, guided assistance using safe-holding skills, you get Sameera onto the ward and hand her over to the nurse in charge.

'You determine that as she is detained under the MHA you should do all you can to persuade, de-escalate and prevent Sameera from absconding.'

Milena

Milena is a 25-year-old female with a history of moderate learning disability.

You are called on scene as Milena has had a bad sprain to her left ankle. She does not wish to go to hospital or have observations done after attempts at persuasion, as she finds crowded spaces very difficult. You determine that Milena does not have capacity. Clinically, you determine that she does not have a life-threatening condition and therefore it is not proportionate to physically intervene. You write up your assessment and have provided a safety net for Milena, referring her onto a primary care colleague and offering worsening advice to an appropriate responsible adult. Following assessment, you may have wanted to take Milena to an emergency department to rule out a fracture and you had identified she lacked capacity. However, the threshold for physical intervention was not proportionate to the presenting risk posed by the potential fracture.

'Clinically, you determine that she does not have a life-threatening condition and therefore it is not proportionate to physically intervene.'

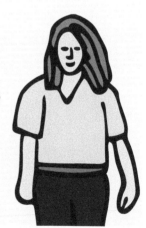

Case studies (continued)

Steve

Steve is a 28-year-old male with a history of emotional difficulties.

You are called to Steve, who has taken a large overdose of amitriptyline with a lot of alcohol. He is agitated and abusive. Steve is a frequent caller and you are aware of a history of aggression towards police and ambulance services. You determine regarding his need for further medical treatment at hospital that Steve does not have capacity, having completed the two-stage test due to alcohol impairment. You have risk assessed and believe Steve is beyond your safe-holding skills for you and your colleague to physically intervene. You are also aware of your duty to preserve life. In this scenario it is appropriate to escalate to police colleagues for support. The following narrative identifies that your request is reasonable and proportionate in relation to the presenting risk to ambulance crews and the patient if he does not receive treatment.

I am an ambulance clinician on scene with a 28-year-old male. The male is reported to have taken a large immediately life-threatening overdose. It is my clinical judgement that the patient lacks capacity due to alcohol temporary impairment. I have risk assessed and due to the likelihood and severity of potential risk of aggression, I believe the patient is beyond my ability to manage safely. Based on his presentation I believe he may die if he is not taken to an emergency department for assessment and treatment. I am requesting your assistance under Section 5 and Section 6 of the Mental Capacity Act 2005. This patient is at high risk of death should he not receive medical intervention.

This conversation needs to be documented as part of the patient clinical record.

'You have risk assessed and believe Steve is beyond your safe-holding skills for you and your colleague.'

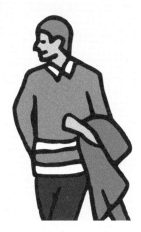

Part 2

Mental Health Conditions Encountered in Prehospital Care

This section includes:

- **Anxiety and Stress**

- **Post-traumatic Stress Disorder**

- **Eating Disorders**

- **Depression**

- **Bipolar Disorder**

- **Psychosis (Schizophrenia)**

- **Personality Disorders**

- **Addiction and Dependence**

Anxiety and Stress

What is anxiety?

Anxiety can be defined as our instinctive physiological and psychological response to a perceived or actual threat. It covers a range of conditions which can involve an emotional state typified by fearfulness, and a collection of associated unpleasant physical symptoms.

Remember, anxiety is a normal human response to a stressful situation. When the levels of anxiety have a significant impact on our functioning it is characterised as unhealthy and therefore a medical condition. Other factors are when it occurs independently of an obvious stressful stimulus, carries on when the stressful stimulus has ceased or is in excess of what would typically be expected from that stressor.

Causes

Patients with a diagnosis of anxiety may have had a traumatic experience in life perhaps related to abuse, neglect, instability or bullying. Stress and anxiety can also be related to sustained unrealistic pressures such as work, finances or family life. People experiencing these conditions often have a lot of internal conflict or conflicting views on decision making. This leads to frequent over-analysis and automatic negative thinking ('glass is always half empty') (Mind, 2021).

Symptoms

Typical symptoms of stress and anxiety include, but are not limited to, the following:

- Poor initial sleep
- Early morning waking
- Shortness of breath
- Palpitations
- Nausea
- Excessive ruminations (constantly overthinking a risk)
- Restlessness / unrealistic fears
  - Heightened alertness
  - Tension in muscles
- Preoccupation
- Difficulty with memory and concentration
- Avoidance
- Irritability
- Frequently needing the toilet
- Change in behaviour
- Clammy hands, dry mouth
- 'Butterflies in tummy'.

Treatment

The most effective form of treatment for anxiety and stress is psychological support, cognitive behavioural therapy (CBT), recovery and resilience work and social support. Medication can be used but ideally on a short-term basis. Some antidepressants can have a positive effect on anxiety management. The main two types are antidepressant classes of drug from the selective serotonin reuptake inhibitor (SSRI) and serotonin-norepinephrine reuptake inhibitor (SNRI) categories. Although medication can have a positive effect, it is important to remember that it often treats the symptoms but not the root cause. This is why medication should be seen as part of a triangulation of treatment to include counselling and social prescribing, which are covered in more detail on page 54 (Mind, 2021).

The amygdala hijack

The amygdala hijack relates to the adrenaline rush and irrational thoughts or behaviour we experience when our threat and self-protection part of the brain is activated. Think about what might trigger this reaction for you. It might be for example spiders, heights or lifts. Think through what is happening in your body. Imagine if you had a more severe, heightened and persistent reaction and how debilitating this could be to your functioning. The chemical reaction below can trigger the irrational fight, flight or freeze response (Goleman, 1996).

We can all have our resilience tested at times. Reflect back to a time when perhaps you or someone you know said or did something they later regretted. Often our resilience or 'bounceability' (see pages 97–98) can be affected in lots of different ways. See the TFL #ShareTheRoad video link on page 26 as an example.

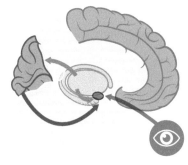

Sensory perception of risk triggers amygdala response

Frontal Lobe
Responsible for memory problem solving and higher cognitive functioning

Occipital Lobe
Visual processing area of the brain

Thalamus
Responsible for some sensory processing such as hearing and seeing

Hippocampus
Plays a major role in learning and memory

Amygdala
Responsible for fearful and threatening stimulus reactions, it also helps define and regulate emotional responses

⊕ Link

For more details on the amygdala hijack, see this useful video from PMSL Training:

▶ https://youtu.be/9u3UvXqArqs

Crisis cycle

The crisis cycle relates to how we can lose reason and objectivity during moments of high stress. In a crisis point, we may say or do things that we later regret upon reflection. Think back to a time where you may have felt overwhelmed and either said or did something you later regretted. It is normal to feel cross or upset when stressed. Understanding the amygdala hijack and crisis cycle, including triggers and helpful coping strategies to prevent escalation, provides us with more opportunity to retain control.

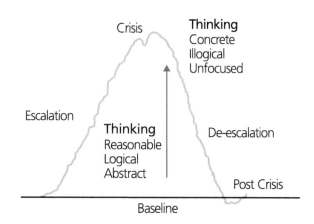

Quick thought

We can all feel cross and angry at times; our resilience can be tested in lots of ways. If there is a build-up of this, there is a risk we can say or do something we later regret. To retain rational objectivity, it is important we reflect on our stress levels and how we can detach to build resilience and self-compassion.

Activity

Signs of anxiety

Map out all the physical and psychological signs and symptoms of anxiety on the body that you are aware of to see the whole impact. Start with two examples: one physical (for example, palpitations) and the second psychological (for example, heightened sense of alertness). Reflect on how these can significantly impact your physical health, psychological health and ability to function effectively.

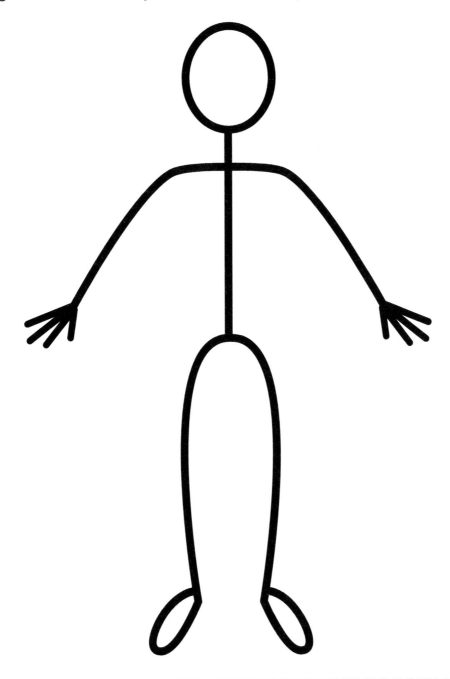

Reflective exercise

Take time to reflect on the impact anxiety can have on both physical and mental health. Can you think of any conditions associated with heightened anxiety which lead to a 999 call?

- For example, Hyperventilation Syndrome 'panic attacks' are often seen by ambulance staff. Patients may become uncontrollably breathless, experience chest pain or unusual sensations in their hands and face or feel faint and weak following a real or perceived emotional stress. The diagnosis of Hyperventilation Syndrome should be one of exclusion, once you are confident that there is no underlying physical pathology after examination and ruling out any medical cause.

Benzodiazepines

Benzodiazepines are a type of sedative that may sometimes be used as a short-term treatment during a particularly severe period of anxiety because they help ease the symptoms within 30 to 90 minutes of taking the medication.

Examples of benzodiazepines you may be prescribed include chlordiazepoxide, diazepam and lorazepam.

Although benzodiazepines are very effective in treating the symptoms of anxiety, they should not be used for long periods of time because they can become addictive if used for longer than four weeks. They also start to lose their effectiveness after this time. For these reasons, patients should not usually be prescribed benzodiazepines for any longer than two to four weeks at a time (NICE, 2014).

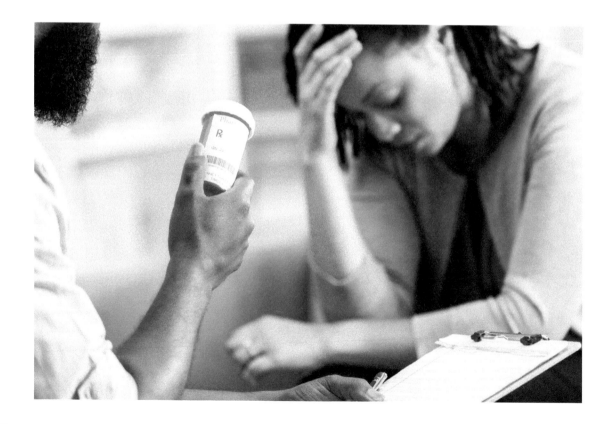

Post-traumatic Stress Disorder

Post-traumatic stress disorder (PTSD) has developed increasing recognition over recent years. The condition can be triggered by any traumatic or perceived traumatic event.

Symptoms

Symptoms can include but are not limited to: nightmares, irritability, guilt, isolation, heightened alertness, anxiety and debilitating flashbacks. The illness was well recognised during World War II, with physicians referring to combat neurosis, combat exhaustion or battle fatigue. In addition to flashbacks, patients may experience an inability to recall, either partially or completely, some important aspects of the period of exposure to the stressor. There may also be persistent symptoms of increased psychological sensitivity and heightened awareness.

Treatment

Treatment of PTSD often includes talking therapies, such as CBT or eye movement desensitisation and reprocessing (EMDR), in the early weeks or months after the event. Whilst some evidence exists to demonstrate the benefit of antidepressant and anxiety medication, the National Institute for Health and Care Excellence (NICE) guidelines do not recommend that this is the first-line treatment (NICE, 2018). Patients often begin to recover with time, although some may have residual symptoms for years after the event.

🌐 Link

For more information regarding PTSD, see the NHS website:

▶ www.nhs.uk/conditions/post-traumatic-stress-disorder-ptsd

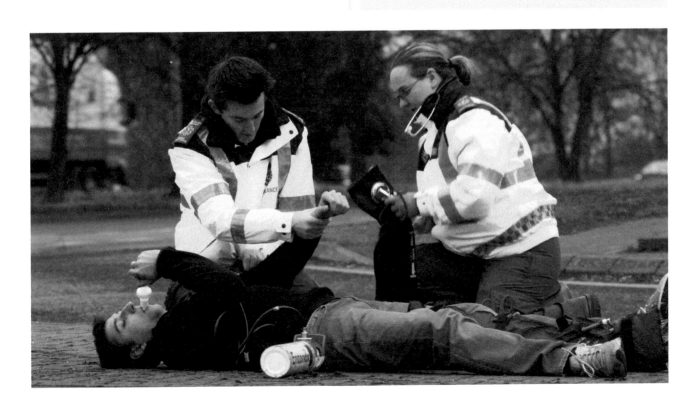

Eating Disorders

This is a broad term for conditions related to anorexia, bulimia and binge eating.

Symptoms

Key symptoms include preoccupation and worrying about weight, low BMI, excessive exercise to control weight, controlling what is eaten or inducing vomiting after eating. Eating disorders can affect men and women of any age but most commonly affects teenagers aged 13–17 years (NHS, 2021).

Treatment

There are a range of talking therapy treatments for eating disorders and it is important to empower the patient to access help via their GP. If there is a significant medical risk related to a dangerously low BMI or physical presentation, you should consult the patient, family, GP and any existing services around safety-netting and treatment.

🌐 Link

For more information regarding eating disorders, see the NHS website:

▶ www.nhs.uk/conditions/eating-disorders

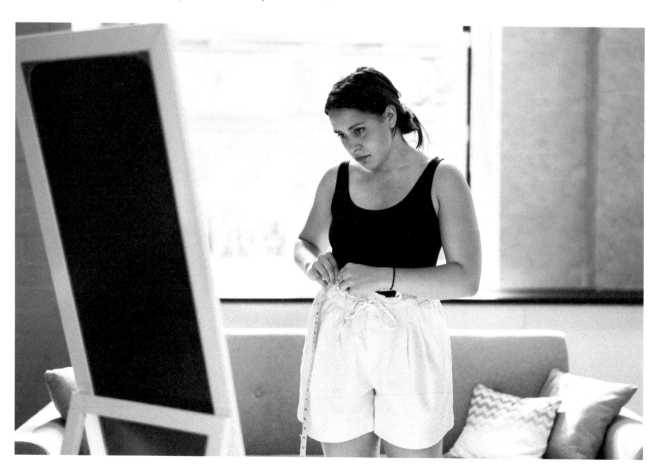

Depression

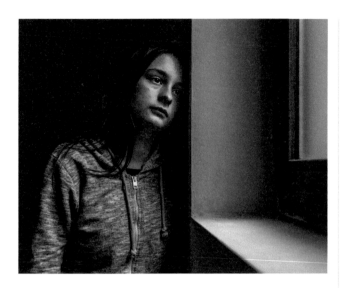

By 2030, depression is projected to become the second greatest cause of 'years lived with disability' worldwide. In the UK, it is estimated that depression affects 5% of adults and 280 million people worldwide. It can also be linked to suicide (World Health Organization, 2021).

Causes

Depression can be triggered by a traumatic life event such as relationship breakup, job loss or bereavement. Of course, anyone can experience grief and low mood in reaction to a loss, but this becomes more of a clinical depressive state when it is severe or sustained. Depression often comes on gradually and many people continue trying to cope without asking for help or even realising they are unwell. There can be a genetic predisposition to a risk of depression, and traumatic early-life experiences can add to vulnerability of experiencing depression. There has been an increase in the prevalence of depression over recent decades. Reasons for this may include changes in society and how we live our lives. Some examples are increased pressure, workload,

social media, expectations, emotional awareness, austerity, social deprivation and a reduction in local extended family contacts (NHS, 2019a).

Symptoms

- Feelings of guilt, worthlessness and hopelessness
- Lack of energy
- Lack of enjoyment in anything
- Sleep disturbance (persistently struggling to get to sleep or early-morning waking)
- Automatic negative thinking (pessimistic)
- Emotional and tearful
- Excessive rumination
- Ambivalence about life and possible thoughts of self-harm
- Change in weight (loss or gain)
- Continuous low mood
- Irritability and intolerance
- Inability to make decisions.

Identifying depression

We can all feel low in mood from time to time related to life events such as financial problems, relationship problems, bereavement or work pressures. For various complex individual reasons, some of us can struggle to bounce back and instead spiral downwards. When the frequency and intensity of the signs and symptoms identified start to have a big impact on our day-to-day functioning (activities of daily living (ADLs)), then it may be reaching a clinical condition. Diagnosing depression can be difficult, especially when it is mild, and patients may be unsure whether their symptoms are simply a natural low mood or are becoming more concerning and need management by their doctor. A diagnosis of depression can only be made via a doctor's examination based on the presenting signs and symptoms.

Some questions you could ask to help referral and signposting are:

1. Do you get little interest or pleasure in doing things?

2. Have you been feeling down, depressed or hopeless in the last month?

3. Have these symptoms been persistent and intense?

4. Are there any recent life events that have seen a change in your mood?

5. Have you or any family or friends noticed a change in you or how you interact?

⊕ Link

'I had a black dog. His name was depression'

https://youtu.be/XiCrniLQGYc

This is a helpful WHO video to outline the signs and symptoms of depression, its impact on functioning and solution-focused approaches.

Treatment

Treatment for long-term or recurrent depression involves psychological approaches such as CBT, social support and efforts to improve lifestyle or functioning (NHS, 2019a). Medication is, however, often a factor in the treatment for more severe depression. It is important that patients consistently take antidepressants. Any gaps in treatment may have a significant impact on the efficacy of antidepressants.

Triangulation of treatment
Treatment & recovery

Social prescribing (ADLs)

Medication   Counselling

Counselling

What is counselling? It is often seen as a therapeutic relationship where you can be open and honest about your thoughts, feelings and behaviour. Structured counselling should be supported by a professional practioner who is independent and unconnected to the patient. The process should be a safe place to be yourself. The counsellor should guide the patient to the key cognitions (thoughts) that are impacting their mood. The main preferred type of counselling in the UK is CBT.

What is CBT?

CBT is based on the premise that thoughts and feelings direct our behaviour. In some people, unhelpful thought processes can lead them to develop negative beliefs about themselves or others, and therefore adopt a pattern of behaviour that perpetuates this, such as isolation and withdrawal. This is summarised in the diagram on page 53.

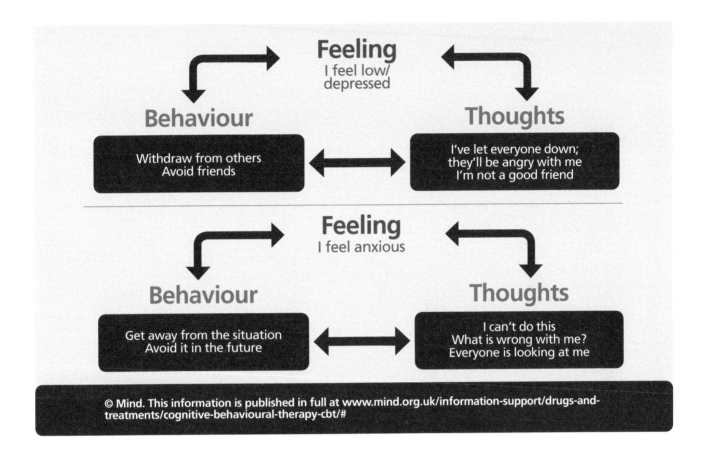

CBT is a talking therapy, undertaken by a specially trained therapist who helps their patient identify which of their thought processes and established beliefs are negative and self-deprecating. From this point, the therapist helps the patient reframe their views to produce behaviour that is positive for them, leading to greater acceptance and solution-focused approaches.

Medication for depression

This section contains lists of classifications of antidepressants and specific examples, starting with the most common. For moderate to severe depression, medication can be effective in some cases but should be determined by the patient and doctor as to suitability or type. Medication for depression should be consistently taken and can take up to six weeks to become clinically effective. Patients should try to avoid alcohol and any illicit drugs whilst on medication as these can be detrimental to treatment. Medication should be seen as a mechanism to treat the symptoms of depression. In order to understand the cause and recovery, medication should be used in combination with counselling and social prescribing to provide the best opportunity for long-term recovery.

Serotonin-specific reuptake inhibitors (SSRIs)

Serotonin-specific reuptake inhibitors (SSRIs), also known as selective serotonin reuptake inhibitors, are usually preferred over other antidepressants as they cause fewer side effects. An overdose is also less likely to be serious.

Fluoxetine is probably the best known SSRI (sold under the brand name Prozac). Other SSRIs include citalopram (Cipramil), paroxetine (Seroxat) and sertraline (Lustral).

Serotonin-noradrenaline reuptake inhibitors (SNRIs)

Serotonin-noradrenaline reuptake inhibitors (SNRIs) are similar to SSRIs. They were designed to be a more effective antidepressant than SSRIs. However, the evidence that SNRIs are more effective in treating depression is uncertain.

It seems some people respond better to SSRIs while others respond better to SNRIs.

Examples of SNRIs include duloxetine (Cymbalta and Yentreve) and venlafaxine (Efexor).

Tricyclic antidepressants (TCAs)

Tricyclic antidepressants (TCAs) are an older type of antidepressant. They are no longer usually recommended as a first-line treatment for depression because they can be more dangerous if an overdose is taken. They also cause more unpleasant side effects than SSRIs and SNRIs.

Exceptions are sometimes made in people with severe depression that fails to respond to other treatments. TCAs may also be recommended for other mental health conditions such as obsessive compulsive disorder and bipolar disorder.

Examples of TCAs include amitriptyline (Tryptizol), clomipramine (Anafranil), imipramine (Tofranil), lofepramine (Gamanil) and nortriptyline (Allegron).

Some types of TCA, such as amitriptyline, can also be used to treat chronic nerve pain.

Monoamine oxidase inhibitors (MAOIs)

Monoamine oxidase inhibitors (MAOIs) are another older type of antidepressant that is rarely used nowadays, with a wide range of side effects. They tend only to be used if other types of antidepressants are not effective, and should only be taken under the supervision of a psychiatrist.

A significant drawback of MAOIs is the need to avoid certain foods and drinks, such as cheese and pickled fish, which contain a protein called tyramine. This is because consuming tyramine while taking MAOIs can cause a dangerous rise in blood pressure.

Examples of MAOIs include moclobemide (Manerix) and phenelzine (Nardil).

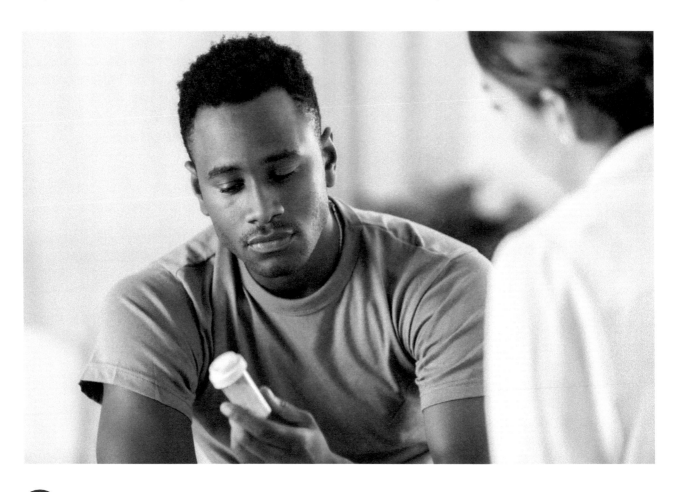

Bipolar Disorder

Bipolar disorder, previously referred to as manic depression, is a condition that relates to significant fluctuations in mood. These manifest as episodes of high mood (mania) and episodes of low mood (depression). Typically, patients will experience an episode for several weeks. Patients in a manic state can be quite vulnerable to making out-of-character decisions and actions that they later regret. Examples of this could include excessive spending, changing jobs or changing relationships.

Symptoms

Mania or hypomania

- Elevated mood
- Rapid speech
- Flight of ideas (constantly changing subject)
- Delusions of grandeur (overly happy, invincible, powerful, important, 'superhuman')
- Excessive spending
- Not sleeping
- Irritability
- Dis-inhibition (out-of-character actions)
- No attention span
- Feeling very creative.

Bipolar depression

- Feelings of guilt, worthlessness and hopelessness
- Lack of energy
- Lack of enjoyment in anything
- Pessimistic
- Emotional and tearful
- Excessive rumination
- Ambivalence about life and possible suicidal thoughts, or thoughts of self-harm

- Change in weight (loss or gain)
- Continuous low mood
- Irritability and intolerance
- Inability to make decisions
- Irrational sleep.

Treatment

The principal aim in treatment of bipolar disorder is overall mood stabilisation, which seeks to level out the peaks of mania and the troughs of depression. This is often achieved using a combination of established medications, many of which were initially developed for alternative medical conditions. Lithium carbonate is one of the most commonly encountered mood stabilising agents, and is normally well tolerated, although the side effects can be significant. Patients occasionally complain of feeling faint and putting on weight, but more serious side effects, which include lithium toxicity (severe gastrointestinal disturbance, drowsiness, ataxia and dysarthria), may be seen.

Other medications commonly used to stabilise mood in bipolar disorder include anticonvulsants, such as sodium valproate and lamotrigine.

In the emergency setting, when patients present with either significant depression or profound mania, the key treatments may include an emergency admission to a psychiatric ward. The decision to admit a patient would need to be made by the existing mental health care or crisis team if known. If not known, this should be considered through a GP. If the patient is deemed to be at high risk to themselves or others following detailed assessment, and is refusing treatment, emergency department or other signposting, then this may require a Mental Health Act assessment via a GP or AMHP.

Psychosis (Schizophrenia)

Psychosis is a severe mental health problem experienced by 1–2% of the population (NHS, 2019c). Often psychosis is thought to be a 'split personality', where the patient possesses and responds to competing personalities. This is, however, an over-simplistic and quite inaccurate description of the diagnosis.

Whilst men and women are affected almost equally, men tend to develop symptoms at an earlier age, often between 19 and 27. There is evidence of a genetic component to psychosis (NHS, 2019c).

Symptoms

Psychosis or schizophrenia leads to alternative or fragmented perceptions of reality. Patients are described as suffering from positive and negative symptoms. In simple terms, positive symptoms 'add' whereas negative symptoms 'take away'.

Positive symptoms include those which are added when the illness is present, such as delusions and hallucinations. Hallucinations are where a person hears, sees, smells or tastes something differently or that is not there. The most common type is auditory hallucinations where patients experience voices, which can be distressing.

Delusions are fixed false beliefs. Typically these can be related to grandiose delusions such as 'believing you are a god' or 'have special powers' or persecutory delusions such as 'being bugged, monitored or followed by the police' or that someone is out to 'harm' them. Negative symptoms are normal feelings or emotions which the disease takes away or dampens, and include apathy, anhedonia, social withdrawal and cognitive delay.

Patients who are psychotic and in crisis can be (but not always) quite impulsive, paranoid and occasionally agitated or aggressive if they feel threatened. Psychotic illnesses can be caused or exacerbated by an excessive use of drugs or alcohol. People with acute or crisis psychotic symptoms require close, careful management due to impulsive risks (NHS, 2019b).

Characteristics of psychosis

- Hallucinations
- Paranoia
- Impulsivity
- Delusions (fixed beliefs)
- Withdrawal and isolation
- Apathetic (emotionless)
- Disorganised thoughts and speech.

Treatment

Patients with a diagnosis of psychosis will often have input from secondary mental health services. They may have a locality community psychiatric nurse (CPN) and are likely to be seen at least twice a year by a consultant psychiatrist as an outpatient. Listed below are common medications that are used in the treatment of psychosis. **It is very important that patients consistently take antipsychotics at the correct prescribed dose, as failure to do so often results in a relapse or deterioration in functioning.**

Modern atypical antipsychotics with fewer side effects include:

- Amisulpride
- Aripiprazole
- Clozapine
- Olanzapine
- Quetiapine
- Risperidone
- Sulpiride.

Older antipsychotics, which cause more side effects but are still used where modern ones are less effective for specific patients, include:

- Chlorpromazine
- Haloperidol
- Pimozide
- Trifluoperazine.

Side effects of antipsychotic medication

Antipsychotic medication (particularly older versions) can have a number of unfortunate side effects, which range from mildly unpleasant through to serious or life-threatening, although this is rare.

At the milder end of the spectrum, patients may complain of sleepiness, slowness, weight gain or impotence. However, rare but more serious side effects include movement disorders such as tardive dyskinesia, long QT syndrome and increased risk of Torsade de Pointes, whereas clozapine can cause bonemarrow suppression leading to neutropenia and severe infection (NICE, 2022).

Recovery

With the right ongoing health and social care support, treatment and engagement, patients with psychosis can go on to have a full recovery. To sustain the recovery, it is important that patients remained engaged with services, continue to consistently take maintenance levels of medication and recognise any potential relapse indicators in order to access help quickly. Having delusions, hallucinations and/or thought disorders can be a very frightening and confusing experience. This is why it is so important to ensure ambulance clinicians have a non-judgemental approach, listen attentively, consider existing care teams and ensure any appropriate new referral is made to a crisis team or that the existing care team is updated if the patient is receiving enhanced support. Further details and information on psychosis can accessed via www.nhs.uk/mental-health/conditions/psychosis/overview/.

Clinical tip

Tardive dyskinesia is a movement disorder of the facial muscles, characterised by lip-smacking, lip-puckering, grimacing and excessive eye movements. It was frequently seen in the past in patients who had taken high dose antipsychotics for many years, although it is seen much less often now due to the advent of modern atypical antipsychotics.

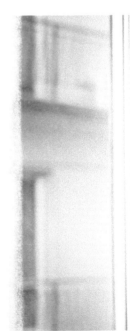
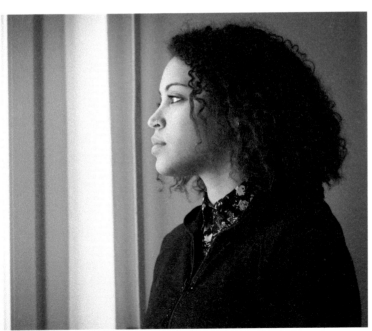

Personality Disorders

In mental health, we frequently use terms that, for us, have an implicit understanding attached to them but if given careful thought are very hard to define. For example, we all innately know what is meant when we speak of consciousness, but if you try to define it and describe what elements are necessary for it to exist, the picture becomes increasingly unclear and confusing! Similarly, when we speak of 'personality', it can be hard to identify exactly what people mean. We all possess a personality, but to define what constitutes a personality is often challenging.

In mental health, 'personality' is commonly described as a collection of characteristics which influence the way in which someone thinks, feels and behaves. Whilst most people have established their personality by their late teens, people with a personality disorder may develop traits in their personality which cause a high degree of emotional distress or internal conflict. This makes it difficult for them to acquire sufficient self-esteem to become resilient to the pressures of normal life. As such, this chronic condition means people think, perceive, relate and feel differently from others.

These personality traits can lead to odd or irrational behaviour which can be distressing and may upset others close to the person.

Symptoms

Personality disorders are often, but not always, triggered by experiences of neglect, abuse or trauma in early developmental life. Symptoms of personality disorder can include:

- Difficulties in forming and maintaining stable close relationships with families, friends, partners and children

- Eccentric, odd or unusual behaviour
- Feelings of distress, anxiety and worthlessness
- Emotional instability and difficulties containing emotional distress
- Difficulties with trust
- History of self-harm or suicidal ideation
- Highly expressed emotions
- Repeated self-harm in adjustment to stressful situations

The frequency of personality disorder in the UK is hard to define, as the diagnostic criteria have undergone a great deal of uncertainty and refinement over the years. Some experts have suggested that as many as one in five people may suffer with a personality disorder, although this estimate is at the extreme end of the spectrum (Royal College of Psychiatrists, 2015). One in twenty might be closer to the true picture (Royal College of Psychiatrists, 2015). Fortunately, and unlike many conditions, personality disorders tend to improve with age.

Treatment

The most effective treatment for patients with a personality disorder is psychological support and psychotherapy (NICE, 2009). No medication is currently licensed for the treatment of any personality disorder. However, medications may be prescribed to treat associated distress or mood problems, such as depression, anxiety and psychotic-type symptoms.

Key reflections for the ambulance service

It can be difficult to support a patient in crisis with a personality disorder. We can often see high levels of emotional distress. It is important to de-escalate as best as possible with a compassionate, non-judgemental approach. Work with the patient on what options they feel would help. Try to reduce or remove any audience or stimulus which is exacerbating the situation, such as distressed families or friends or loud music. Focus on immediate positive options and solutions. Provide choices and outcomes on what would help reduce levels of distress, empowering the patient to contribute and find solutions.

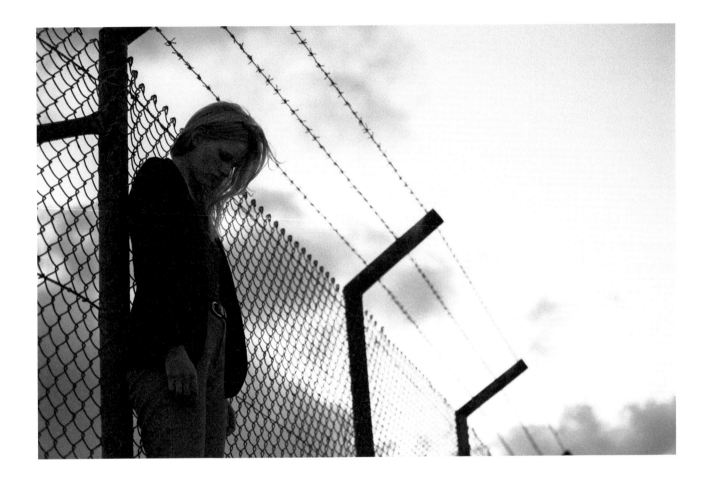

Addiction and Dependence

There are often complex reasons why a patient may have developed a dependence on drugs or alcohol. It is important to understand the frequency, intensity and impact on physical and mental health of any dependency. Patients often describe levels of stigma and pre-conceived ideas around dependence. This is why it is important to build a therapeutic rapport, to have a non-judgemental approach and to work with the patient to establish the right course of action, based on potential risks and available pathways.

Drug and alcohol dependence are more prevalent in urban areas, with data showing cities such as Brighton, Cardiff and Liverpool as having some of the highest levels of drug misuse (Delamere, 2021).

As any clinician who has worked in frontline ambulance duties will know, drug use in the UK is common and on the increase. Many patients cite drug use as a way to block out distress related to past trauma and abuse.

Alcohol

Alcohol misuse is a growing problem in the UK; the burden on healthcare systems is increasing, and the cost to society is unquestionable. There are an estimated 586,780 dependent drinkers in England and there were 9,214 alcohol-related deaths in 2016 (Alcohol Change UK, 2021). Alcohol misuse rates are commonly higher amongst those from lower social-economic backgrounds and in homeless populations (Alcohol Change UK, n.d.). In addition to the physical damage that alcohol abuse can cause, it also exacerbates the severity and frequency of depressive, psychotic and anxiety-related symptoms in those with a diagnosed mental health problem.

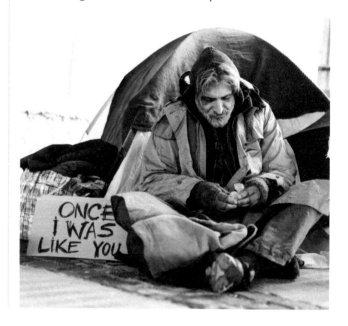

Clinical tip:
Key terminology in substance misuse

Harmful use
A pattern of drug or alcohol misuse that incurs either physical or mental harm to the user. Examples include alcoholic liver disease or acute psychosis.

Dependence syndrome
Dependence on drugs or alcohol is characterised by a triad of diagnostic features. The patient demonstrates a compulsion to use the substance which takes priority over everything else in their life.

Tolerance to the substance is when a gradually increasing amount is required to attain the same effect.

Withdrawal may occur, whereby the user suffers physical and mental symptoms when the substance is not available.

🌐 Link

In 2018, there were 7,551 alcohol-related deaths in the UK. Two-thirds of these deaths were amongst men. More information, statistics and discussion can be found on the Office for National Statistics' website (https://www.ons.gov.uk/).

Managing drug and alcohol addiction

The treatment of drug and alcohol dependence is detoxification, normally via a community or inpatient programme. A variety of pharmaceutics are available to alleviate withdrawal symptoms, manage anxiety and improve physical health.

However, underpinning these approaches are various individual and group therapies which help service users identify the trigger for their addiction, and build more suitable coping strategies for the future.

Ambulance clinicians generally have very little involvement in the chronic management of patients with an addiction, and more frequently encounter them during a mental health crisis or a physical overdose. There are established protocols available to guide the management of overdose of alcohol and drugs within the JRCALC clinical guidelines. When the patient's need is more aligned to mental health services, it is important to establish which professionals are already involved in the patient's care, and use these as a point of reference wherever possible. In some circumstances where there is a potential high risk of harm or medical condition, it may be necessary to consider capacity, decision making and risk management.

Clinical tip: Detecting alcohol misuse

It can be difficult to detect whether a patient is suffering from an undiagnosed alcohol dependency, sometimes because the patient may not recognise it themselves. One helpful screening tool available to ambulance clinicians is the **CAGE (Cut, Annoyed, Guilty, Eye)** mnemonic (Ewing, 1984).

1. Have you ever felt you should **Cut** down on your drinking?

2. Have people **Annoyed** you by criticising your drinking?

3. Have you ever felt bad or **Guilty** about your drinking?

4. Have you ever had an **Eye-opener** drink first thing in the morning to steady your nerves or get rid of a hangover?

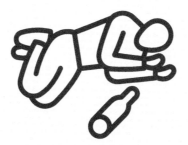

Part 3

Complex Needs

This section includes:

- Learning Disabilities

- Autism and Neurodiversity

- Dementia

Learning Disabilities

There are approximately 1.5 million people living with a learning disability in the UK (Foundation for People with Learning Disabilities, 2021). People with learning disabilities should be able to expect high-quality care across all services provided by the NHS. They should receive treatment, care and support that is safe and personalised. They should have access to the same services and outcomes as their non-disabled peers.

What is a learning disability?

A learning disability is very individual and will be different for everyone that has one. Someone with a learning disability may have a reduced intellectual ability and due to this they may have difficulty with everyday activities or expressing their needs (Mencap, n.d.). This could be problems managing household tasks, budgeting, socialising or managing their own health. A learning disability is lifelong.

People with a learning disability can take longer to learn and may need support to develop new skills. With the right help, they can often lead independent lives. The level of support someone needs depends on the individual. For example, someone with a mild learning disability may only need support with things like getting a job. However, someone with a severe or profound learning disability may need full-time care and support with every aspect of their life – they may also have physical health problems.

There are different types of learning disability, which can be mild, moderate or severe. A person may have difficulties such as:

- Mobility issues or physical disability
- Problems managing their own personal care
- Communication difficulties
- Problems managing their own safety
- Difficulty making their own decisions or problem solving.

What causes a learning disability?

Several things, can cause a learning disability. A learning disability occurs when the brain is still developing (before, during or soon after birth).

- Before birth, things can happen to the central nervous system (the brain and spinal cord) that can cause a learning disability. A child can be

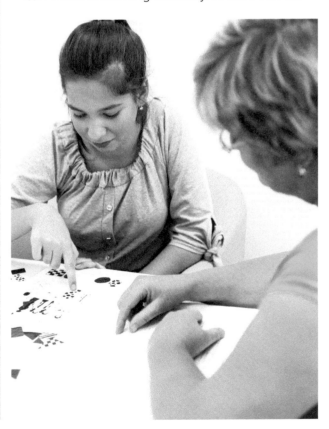

born with a learning disability if the mother has an accident or illness while she is pregnant, or if the unborn baby develops certain genes (NHS, 2022).

- During birth, a person can be born with a learning disability if they do not get enough oxygen during childbirth, have trauma to the head or are born too early.

- After birth, a learning disability can be caused by early childhood illnesses, accidents and seizures up to the age of 18 years.

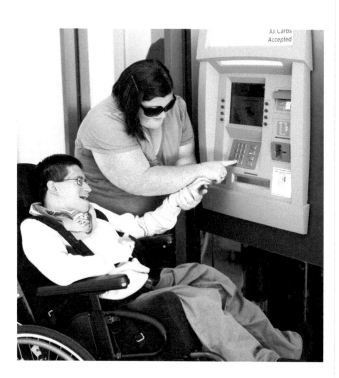

What can be confused for a learning disability?

Autism

Like a learning disability, autism is a lifelong condition. It has three features that might affect the way a person:

1. Interacts with others in a social situation

2. Is able to communicate with others

3. Thinks about and deals with social situations.

Autism is not a learning disability, but around half of the people with autism also have a diagnosed learning disability (Foundation for People with Learning Disabilities, 2022). There is more information about autism on pages 71–75.

Asperger syndrome

Asperger syndrome, also known as Asperger's, is a form of autism which may affect the way a person relates to others and communicates. People with Asperger syndrome may have anxiety, or a specific learning difficulty such as dyslexia. People with Asperger's have an average or above average intelligence and therefore have no learning disability.

Mild learning difficulties

Specific mild learning difficulties may include:

- **Dyslexia** – A problem with written language
- **Dyscalculia** – A problem with numbers
- **Dysgraphia** – Inability to write
- **Dyspraxia** – Difficulty in co-ordinating movement.

Medical complications

People with learning disabilities tend to die at a younger age than the general population. On average, the life expectancy of women with a learning disability is 17 years shorter than for women in the general population; the life expectancy of men with a learning disability is 14 years shorter than for men in the general population (NHS Digital, 2020b). Reports by Mencap show that inadequate care is a cause of some of the deaths amongst this population (Mencap, 2007).

In June 2015, the Learning Disabilities Mortality Review Programme (also known as LeDeR) was established. The aim of the project is to make improvements to the lives of people with learning disabilities. It clarifies any potentially modifiable factors associated with a person's death, and works to ensure that these are not repeated elsewhere.

A number of barriers stop people with a learning disability from receiving good healthcare, leading to poor outcomes. These barriers include:

- A lack of accessible transport links
- Patients not being identified as having a learning disability
- Staff having little understanding about learning disabilities
- Failure to recognise that a person with a learning disability is unwell
- Failure to make a correct diagnosis
- Anxiety or a lack of confidence in people with a learning disability
- Lack of joint working from different care providers
- Not enough involvement allowed from carers
- Inadequate aftercare or follow-up care.

(Hosking et al., 2016; Rickard and Donkin, 2018)

Communication

People with learning disabilities often have problems with communication. Every person is an individual and their needs will be different. It is important to check what works best for the person.

Tips for better communication

- Find an appropriate place to talk without distractions
- Ask open questions
- Check the person understands by using appropriate paraphrasing. For example, 'you felt sick, is that right?'.

Reflective exercise

Try to imagine:

- Not being able to read this
- Not being able to tell someone else about it
- Not being able to find the words you want to say
- Opening your mouth and no sound coming out
- Words coming out jumbled up
- Not getting the sounds right
- Words getting stuck, and someone jumping in and saying words for you
- People assuming what you want, without checking with you
- Not hearing the questions
- Not being able to see, or not being able to understand the signs and symbols around you
- Not understanding the words, phrases or expressions
- Not being able to write down your ideas
- Being unable to join a conversation
- People ignoring what you're trying to say, feeling embarrassed and moving away
- People not waiting long enough for you to respond in some way, assuming you have nothing to say and moving away.

(Mencap, 2018)

69

- If a person wants to take you to show you something, go with them

- Keep a keen eye for non-verbal communication such as body language, gestures and facial expression

- Take time; do not rush things

- Use everyday language at every opportunity

- Look for support from carers or family who know and understand communication needs.

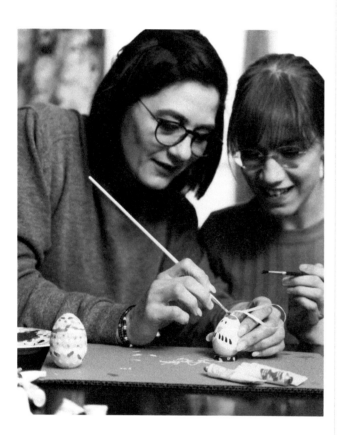

Legal issues
Mental Capacity Act

The Mental Capacity Act is an important law for people with learning disabilities. It protects an individual's right to make their own choices and gives others the duty to make decisions if the person is not able to. Please refer back to the Legal Framework and Decision Making section on pages 34–43 for more information about the Mental Capacity Act.

Just like the general population, people with a learning disability may or may not need an assessment of their mental capacity to provide treatment or transportation to hospital.

Reasonable adjustments

Reasonable adjustments are a legal duty under the Equality Act (2010) and must be made by health services to help people with learning disabilities access services. Reasonable adjustments ensure a person with a learning disability gets as good a service as everyone else. The adjustments should be individual for the person needing the support.

Some examples of reasonable adjustments are:

- Easy-to-read information

- Allocating more time for appointments

- Using everyday communication

- Reading and acting on information given in communication passports, hospital traffic light assessments or care plans.

Every person is an individual and their needs will be different; it is important to check what works best for the person.

Autism and Neurodiversity

What is autism and what is neurodiversity?

Autism is a lifelong neurodevelopmental condition. It is not a disability or an impairment but a difference in brain configuration resulting in a different way that information is cognitively processed. Understanding these differences is important to improve patient experience of the ambulance service. Autism has been described as 'a relatively common neurodevelopmental condition, usually associated with normal IQ range, that represents a form of natural variation, bringing both strengths and challenges' (Mandy, 2018).

Autism is one example of what we understand to be a hidden form of natural human variation, now known as neurodiversity. The notion behind the concept of neurodiversity is that brain differences are normal and to be expected, rather than deficits. This stance can help reduce stigma as well as improving engagement around learning and thinking differences. Most people are described as neurologically typical (or neurotypical), meaning that their brains function and process information in the way 'society expects'.

Neurodivergence is a relatively new term that includes autism, attention deficit disorder, dyslexia and dyspraxia and other neurological conditions. These are 'spectrum' conditions, with a wide range of characteristics, that share some common features in terms of how people learn and process information. This results in neurodivergent individuals having different experiences of the world around them and interacting with the world in a different way. Although these differences can pose a challenge for the neurodivergent population, a world with neurodiversity brings additional talents that are essential for the development of humankind.

1–2 % of the UK population are known to be autistic (NHS Digital, 2020a). However, this is likely to be an underestimate due to difficulties in obtaining diagnosis for autism and many autistic people successfully living with autism that will not feel the need to pursue a diagnosis.

Whilst there are a lot of claims about the cause of autism, these are unsupported and autism is not the result of MMR vaccination, diet, vitamin deficiency, pollution or upbringing.

Differences in cognitive processing

There are key differences in the way an autistic brain processes information, outlined below.

Sensory

The world around us is full of constant sensory information being received to our brain; in non-autistic brains most of this information is filtered out.

In autism, we see this filtering as not working in the same way; autistic people can receive too much sensory information (hyper-sensitivity) or too little sensory information (hyposensitivity). This key difference results in very different experiences of the world and places additional demands on cognitive processing capacity.

At times this can be extremely distracting for the person and can lead to periods of feeling completely overwhelmed by the amount of information being processed.

Monotropism

Monotropism describes an information processing style where singular parts of information are initially viewed and processed individually, with these various separate pieces of information then being connected to form the bigger picture. Monotropism contrasts with polytropism, where all the information is processed simultaneously to instantly create the bigger picture although often detail is missed. Polytropism is the usual processing style for the 'neurotypical' population. Neither style is dysfunctional or impaired, they are simply different ways of looking at the same information – one in more specific detail, the other with a broader perspective. A better understanding of monotropism can highlight some key differences seen in autistic people:

- **Strong attention to detail**: Autistic people have an enhanced ability to spot patterns and omissions within complex data.

- **Literal use of social language**: Autistic people tend to interpret the exact, literal meaning of words or phrases. Our social world can be confusing for autistic people as we often say what we do not explicitly mean and frequently use idioms and metaphors which if taken at face value become confusing (for example, 'pull your socks up' is a common phrase that can be interpreted very differently when considered literally).

- **Executive functioning**: This is the cognitive processes that support us to achieve our goals and manage our complex lives; planning, sequencing, prioritising, organising can be challenging for autistic people as multiple simultaneous cognitive processes are required in these areas.

Autism diagnosis

These key differences in cognitive processing explain the outward presentation we see in autistic people. It is the outward differences that lead to diagnosis being made by suitably trained and qualified professionals. Differences in social communication and interaction, repetitive behaviours and strong interests in the context of developmental history provide the diagnosis of autism.

More males than females are currently diagnosed with autism (Loomes, Hull and Mandy, et al., 2017). However, current assessments are based on a male autistic presentation, and autism in females presents differently and can be more subtle.

Signs of autism in adults

Not all autistic people are the same, in the same way that not all neurotypical or non-autistic people are the same. Below are some common signs of autism in adults that may present on clinical assessment in prehospital care:

- Seeming blunt, rude or disinterested in others without meaning to, this can include not giving eye contact.

- Finding it difficult to communicate your emotions.

- Becoming anxious about social situations.

- Having the same routine every day and getting very anxious if it changes.

- Liking to plan events carefully before they happen.

- Understanding things in a very literal sense, for example, may not understand sarcasm.

- Difficulty understanding what others are thinking or feeling.

- Difficulty making and maintaining friendships.

(NHS, 2019)

Having an awareness of these can improve communication and build rapport, ultimately enabling engagement and providing choices.

Challenges faced by neurodivergent people

Autism (and neurodiversity) is not a problem and should not be a disadvantage; it is another form of naturally occurring biodiversity, much like ethnicity, sexuality or even being left handed. However, research tells us that autistic people have poorer health outcomes (Doherty et al., 2022; Bishop-Fitzpatrick and Kind, 2017), and studies have suggested that the risk of early mortality in the autistic population than non-autistic population is anywhere between two and ten times greater (Guan and Li, 2017). Individuals with autism are also nine times more likely to die by suicide (Autistica, n.d.).

The challenge for autistic individuals is our world is currently set up for one type of cognitive typical functioning. It is very much like being an Apple Mac laptop in a world of Microsoft where your laptop is expected to work well on Microsoft software. The difference in functioning and needs are not accommodated.

Autistic people can prefer routines and predictability; knowing what is happening next is reassuring and decreases anxiety yet we live in a highly unpredictable and unstructured world. Communication, if not clear, concise and unambiguous can become misleading and confusing. The sensory world can also pose a big challenge; imagine being badly affected by certain types of lighting and certain types of sounds that can cause you acute distress, yet these sensory challenges are forever present as no-one else is affected by them.

These are challenges we have probably all faced at some point but for neurodiverse individuals these are daily, constant challenges that become tiring and exhausting.

Supporting an autistic person in prehospital medical or mental health crisis care

When overwhelmed by the sensory and social world around them and the complex demands of everyday living, autistic people can experience extreme psychological distress leading to the person experiencing meltdown or shut down. These are extreme fight, flight or freeze responses described under the amygdala hijack section of this workbook (page 48).

- Autistic people may wear a sunflower lanyard, this is informing you of a hidden form of diversity.

- Consider the sensory environment (blue lights, sirens, radios, ambulance layout or other sensory environment factors) – the person may be experiencing sensory overload.

- If someone is in meltdown or shut down, they will benefit from being supported to a quiet, calm area with less stimulus and ideally dull lighting. They may benefit from being alone, so if you need to be there to support or assess try reducing verbal communication and interaction until they are ready to receive this.

- Be very mindful of providing physical touch to reassure an autistic person, as many autistic people can find touch to be difficult. If you do need to apply physical touch to carry out any observations, it is a good idea to inform the person first.

Communication with an autistic person

- Be positive about autism: use language of difference, not disability; do not describe the person as suffering with autism; be interested in their lived experience and them as an individual.

73

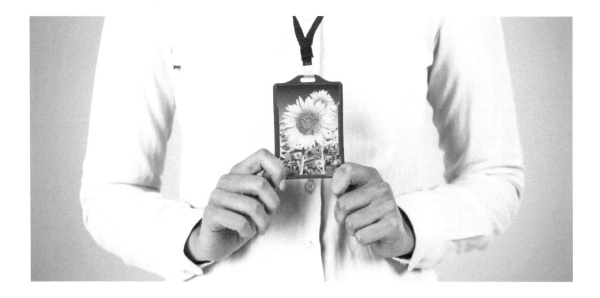

- Use the person's name to gain attention and focus.

- Do not expect eye contact; their focus is your words, not you.

- Allow time for the person to process the information and respond; our uncomfortable silence is an autistic person processing time.

- Use clear, concise language and say exactly what you meant. Avoid using idioms, metaphors and sarcastic humour.

- Be predictable: clearly outline next steps or intended actions and deliver this as expected; if several steps are required list these in order of completion.

- Emphasise key pieces of information that should be remembered.

- Avoid open-ended questions: use forced-choice or closed questioning style.

- If you are a control room call-taker, consider whether a clinician would be more appropriate to take the call as they do not have to utilise the NHS pathways or medical priority dispatch system (MPDS) logarithm process.

Need for adjustment

As autism is about a diverse form of brain function there is no treatment or cure, we are not going to change the person. Autism requires our understanding and acceptance and for us to do things differently to accommodate and include the needs of our autistic population.

This is a legal requirement under the Equality Act 2010 where autism (and other neurodiversity) are recognised protected characteristics, entitling the person to reasonable adjustments. As you would when communicating with all vulnerable people in prehospital care, take time to adapt your clinical practice to meet the needs of the person and the nature of emergency call.

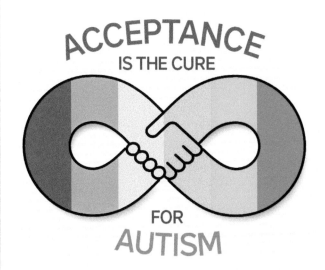

Reasonable adjustment concept for autism

The following adjustments are recommended for consideration:

- Acceptance: A culture of acceptance and understanding of autism and that adjustments are needed to reduce barriers to access.

- Predictability: Uncertainty and lack of predictability are anxiety provoking. We will make our emergency service pathways and settings as predictable as possible.

- Information: Information and detail help provide context and build the bigger. We will communicate information that is clear, concise and explicit.

- Processing: Anxiety and sensory distractions will impact on processing. We will use supplementary materials (such as diagrams or text) to support the processing of verbal information.

- Sensory: Environments with challenging sensory stimuli will impact on processing and can lead to person being overwhelmed. We will be mindful of visual stimuli (bright or blue lights), noise (background noises and sirens), odours (perfumes, aftershaves and cleaning products) and remove these where possible.

⊕ Link

Amazing Things Happen!: Introduction to Autism

▶ https://youtu.be/Ezv85LMFx2E

Dementia

Did you know there are around 900,000 people living with dementia in the UK (Alzheimer's Society, 2021)? Dementia is an umbrella term used to describe a range of progressive conditions affecting the brain. There are over 200 subtypes of dementia, but the 5 most common are: Alzheimer's disease, vascular dementia, dementia with Lewy bodies, frontotemporal dementia and mixed dementia. 'Mixed dementia' is the term commonly used if a person has a combination of different types of dementia (Dementia UK, 2021).

Other, rarer causes of dementia exist such as Creutzfeldt-Jakob disease (CJD), but these are very often seen in isolated cases, and the general principles of assessment and referral used in the more common dementias are applicable to these patients also.

An important step in recognising dementia is increasing public understanding that a significant decline in cognitive function is not part of the normal process of ageing. Indeed, many of the symptoms of early dementia might be considered as 'normal' in the ageing adult, and for this reason, the diagnosis can be missed or made very late.

Delays in dementia diagnosis can be due to a number of factors, including difficulty diagnosing in the early stages and the slow progression and limited public awareness of the diseases that cause dementia (Dementia UK, 2021). A delay in diagnosis can mean the person and their family are not aware of or able to access the support that is available to people affected by dementia.

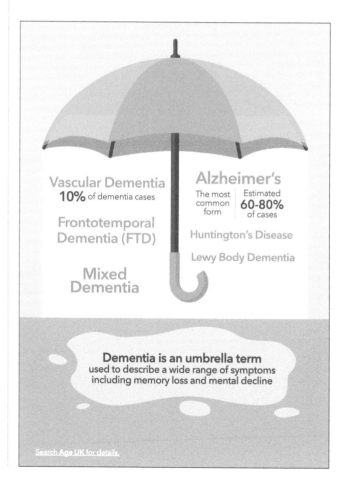

Vascular Dementia
10% of dementia cases

Frontotemporal Dementia (FTD)

Mixed Dementia

Alzheimer's
The most common form | Estimated **60-80%** of cases

Huntington's Disease

Lewy Body Dementia

Dementia is an umbrella term
used to describe a wide range of symptoms including memory loss and mental decline

Search Age UK for details.

Activity

Dementia or normal ageing?

Complete the table below, putting the symptoms of dementia and ageing into their appropriate boxes; where they apply to both processes, place them across the centre.

Dementia	Both	Normal ageing

Symptoms:

Uncharacteristic agitation

Impaired judgement

Difficulty with abstract thought

Withdrawal

Isolation

Forgetting where they left the car

Forgetting some words in a sentence

Muddling words up when speaking

Mood changes

Forgetting people's names

Forgetting where they left the car keys

Personality changes

Fluctuations in consciousness

Changes in gait and posture

Incontinence

Disinhibition

Getting confused in unfamiliar places

Hopefully the activity on page 76 will help outline just how difficult it can be for patients, family members and even clinicians to decide if the patient is displaying the normal signs of ageing, so-called 'age-related cognitive decline', or has a pathological process such as dementia. Dementia is not a natural part of ageing and although it is much more common in people over the age of 65, it does not just affect older people. Over 42,000 people under 65 in the UK have young-onset dementia (Alzheimer's Society UK, 2021).

Symptoms

Commonly, the early symptoms of dementia are very subtle, and it may just be a feeling from the patient or the family member that things are not quite right. They may describe:

- Memory loss – especially problems with memory for recent events, such as forgetting messages, routes or names

- Asking questions repetitively

- Increasing difficulties with tasks and activities that require organisation and planning

- Becoming confused in unfamiliar environments

- Difficulty finding the right words

- Difficulty with numbers and/or handling money

- Changes in personality and mood

- Depression

- Periods of being alert or drowsy, or fluctuating levels of confusion

- Visual hallucinations

- Becoming slower than expected in their physical movements

- Becoming less sensitive to other people's emotions, perhaps making them seem cold and unfeeling

- Loss of some inhibitions, leading to behaviour that is out of character, such as making tactless or inappropriate comments.

Types of dementia

The type of dementia that the patient is developing often influences the physical manifestations of the disease, and once a diagnosis is obtained, the clusters of symptoms a person may experience as their dementia progresses can often be predicted. As an example, people with frontotemporal dementia have language problems and behavioural problems, as these functions are associated with the frontal lobes of the brain, which are typically affected by this type of dementia. They may not speak, or may speak in shorter sentences. They may appear distant or rude in conversation.

Patients with vascular dementia may have multiple small infarcts within the vasculature of the brain, which means they can experience symptoms sometimes seen in transient ischaemic attacks, such as confusion, dysphasia and unusual sensations. Their decline is often described as 'stepwise', as they never quite regain the function they had after each small infarct. Other patients with vascular dementia may experience little bleeds in their brain caused by small vessel disease, which leads to localised damage throughout the brain.

Patients with Alzheimer's disease typically suffer from lapses in short-term memory, especially early in the disease, as the protein plaques characteristic of the condition initially attack the hippocampus. This can lead to difficulties in day-to-day function where short-term memory is vital, such as shopping and managing administrative affairs. As dementia progresses, memory loss and difficulties with communication often become very severe. In the later stages, the person is likely to neglect their own health and require constant care.

People with advanced dementia may not recognise close family and friends, remember where they live or know where they are. They may find it impossible to process simple pieces of information, carry out basic tasks or follow instructions.

As dementia progresses, it is common for people to have increasing difficulty speaking and they may eventually lose the ability to speak altogether.

It is important to keep trying to communicate with people with advanced dementia and to recognise and use other, non-verbal means of communication, such as body language, gestures, facial expression and, when appropriate, touch.

Bladder incontinence in the later stages of dementia is common and some people will also experience bowel incontinence. They may be at risk of self-neglect and require increasing support with their activities of daily living.

Management

Until recently, the management of dementia focused almost entirely on helping relatives manage behaviour that was seen as challenging and providing support to the patient, especially through optimising their physical health. Whilst supporting the person and their loved ones still remains important, the biggest recent advancement in dementia care has arguably been the advent of acetylcholinesterase inhibitors (donepezil, galantamine and rivastigmine) for mild to moderate Alzheimer's disease (and certain other types of dementia). Although these medications cannot reverse the pathological changes associated with the diseases, they can ease symptoms and slow down the progression of the disease for a while for some people, enabling patients and their families to have a greater quality of life for a longer period.

Unfortunately, there is currently no cure for any of the diseases that cause dementia. Researchers all over the world are looking for ways to prevent and treat dementia. Meanwhile, the provision of person-centred care can help individuals to live well with dementia.

A person with dementia may have a 'This is me' or 'Knowing me' document where you can find out more about their individual needs and preferences. These documents are the property of the person with dementia and should travel with them if they are being conveyed to hospital.

Key reflections

Unlike functional mental health problems (such as depression), dementia relates to traumatic injury or degeneration of the organ of the brain rather than cognitive functioning. All types of dementia are progressive and regressive, meaning that the condition gets worse over time and that patients typically regress to earlier memories, sometimes not recognising people close to them. Dementia affects the individual and those around them, and both the person and their loved ones may need support to live well with dementia.

From an ambulance perspective, it is important to focus on the here and now and engage with the person in a compassionate, solution-focused way. Unfamiliar situations can be distressing for people with dementia, so using the patient's preferred name, explaining who you are and what is happening and then repeating this information as often as required may be helpful. It is important to involve the person and their carers as much as possible to find solutions that meet their individual needs.

Case study – Doris

You attend to Doris who is 85 years old with moderate dementia and a suspected UTI. Doris seems confused, anxious, distressed, in a state of neglect and is looking for her husband Fred. You are aware from a relative that Fred sadly died two years earlier. Rather than reminding Doris of this fact, you redirect the conversation to focus on being there to help, getting a warm drink and any opportunities to de-escalate or reduce stimulus and levels of distress. This may involve contacting a family member (or friend) who knows Doris well, if appropriate. You carry out an examination, seek clarity from family or friends and treat, signpost or convey Doris according to risks.

Every condition, and the clinical management of the condition, is decision specific and scenario based proportionate to presenting risk. This includes suitable treatment options and protecting the rights or wishes of the patient. Using your clinical judgement and balancing the least restrictive options with a positive duty of care, think through some of the questions below in relation to Doris' case study.

- Is there a concern about balancing medical need and capacity to consent?

- If Doris is assessed to lack capacity, what is the least restrictive treatment option and what is in Doris' best interests?

- Is there a need for ongoing social care support and discussion with a GP about the possible alternatives to hospital?

- Are there any safeguarding concerns and what could these be?

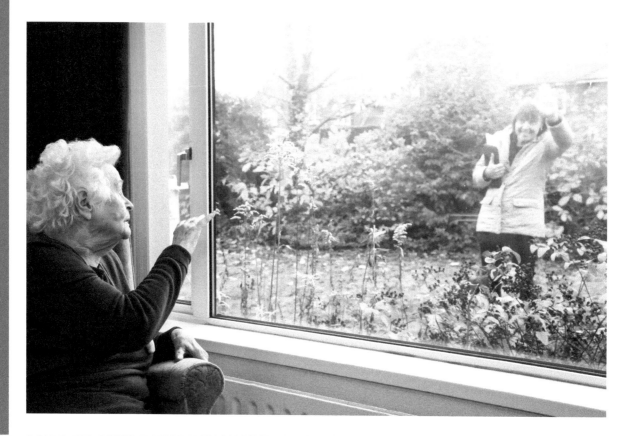

Case study – Doris (continued)

🌐 Link

You may find the link below helpful if you wish to learn more about the various types of dementia, from the Alzheimer's Society, 'Key publications about dementia':

▶ www.alzheimers.org.uk/site/scripts/documents_info.php?documentID=2578

Part 4

Suicide and Self-harm

This section includes:

- **Understanding Suicide**

- **Risk Factors**

- **Risk Management**

- **Self-harm**

Understanding Suicide

Suicide is a very tragic, difficult and emotive subject. Please do seek support if you have professionally or in your personal life experienced suicide which has had a lasting impact on your thoughts or emotions.

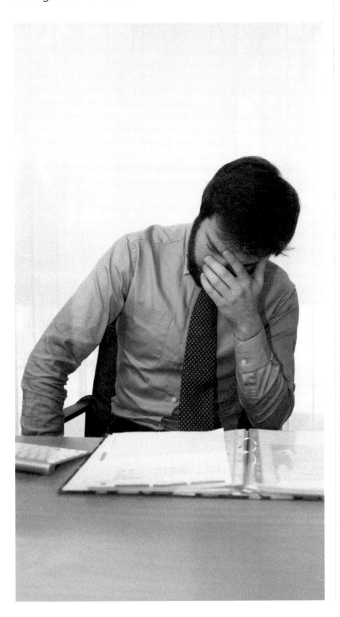

Suicide is a leading cause of death in both developed and developing countries. In England and Wales, there were 5,691 suicides in 2019 which is an increase from 5,420 in 2018 (Office for National Statistics, 2020). Of these, over 75% were men. Evidence suggests the higher rates in men partially relate to perceived weakness and stigma around talking about mental health.

In 2007, the suicide rate had declined to a historic low; however, rates have been rising since 2008, with the recession and austerity cited as possible causes (Healthcare Quality Improvement Partnership, 2021). Similarly, in 2020 the Royal College of Psychiatrists predicted an increase in mental health conditions, particularly in young people and children, as a result of the difficult and unique challenges of the global COVID-19 pandemic and the ensuing social and economic impacts (Royal College of Psychiatrists, 2021). As we have already highlighted, the suicide rate is now growing, and poses a genuine public health concern. Prehospital clinicians are therefore very likely to meet patients who have tried to take their life, and having some understanding of how to approach this situation is key to providing the best care for your patient.

Evidence suggests that over 80% of patients who die by suicide have had a diagnosis of a mental health condition (Mental Health First Aid England, 2020). Many of the remaining 20% will have had difficulties with relationships, finances, addiction, work, social circumstances or trauma (Mental Health Foundation, 2021a). It is therefore imperative that in dealing with any patient who has, or you suspect may have, a mental illness or social crisis, you directly include an evaluation of their suicide risk as part of your assessment.

Risk Factors

What might make someone think of suicide?

It is difficult to predict exactly who may be at risk of suicide but if people seem down or hopeless it is always best to start with a compassionate conversation. People will consider suicide for different reasons; some risk factors might include:

- Difficult life events, such as a traumatic childhood or experiencing physical, sexual, emotional or domestic abuse
- Life-changing situations, such as a relationship ending, a loved one dying, loss of job or siblings moving out
- Anger at other people
- Misusing drugs or alcohol
- Isolation, living alone or having little social contact with other people
- Feeling like they have no friends
- Having a mental health condition such as depression, anxiety, schizophrenia or personality disorder
- Having a physical health condition, especially if this causes pain or serious disability
- Problems with work or money
- Being bullied
- Feelings of hopelessness and helplessness.

When dealing with individuals with suicide ideation, we should assess each case on its own merits and respond according to circumstances and presentation.

This guidance does not change practitioners' current legal duties of confidentiality in respect to the people they are working with. The guidance is designed to support practitioners faced with concerning situations where a patient is suggesting or showing signs that they may end their life.

Warning signs

As practitioners, it is important to have some training to understand the warning signs of someone feeling suicidal. For example, a change in someone's personality and behaviour might be a sign that they are having suicidal thoughts. Often those who know the person are the best judges of when someone is behaving differently. Changes to look out for can include someone:

- Becoming anxious
- Being more irritable
- Being more confrontational
- Becoming quiet and distracted
- Having mood swings
- Acting recklessly
- Sleeping too much or too little
- Changing their eating habits
- Not wanting to be around other people and withdrawing from friends or family members
- Avoiding contact with friends or family
- Having problems with work or studies
- Saying negative things about themselves
- Believing they are a burden and people are better off without them
- Not responding to praise.

Key indicators that suggest someone is more likely to attempt suicide include when they are:

- Threatening to hurt or kill themselves
- Giving verbal hints such as 'I won't be a problem much longer'
- Talking or writing about death, dying or suicide
- Preparing to end their life (for example, by storing up medication, putting their affairs in order, giving away belongings, writing a suicide note or making a will).

Asking about suicide

There is a common misconception that asking a patient about whether they have considered suicide may in some way suggest to them that this is an option. This is entirely false, and there is no evidence to support this theory. By asking the question in a compassionate and confidential way, you provide the opportunity for a patient to open up to a professional if suicide is a risk. By directly asking, you can also understand the level of risk and how to appropriately and proportionately escalate or safeguard. Think about intent, plan, access to means and protective factors or lack of (IPAP) or your organisation's risk-screening tools as per ambulance service guidelines and patient record forms.

Activity

Asking about suicide

What questions might you choose to ask your patient, to give you a better understanding of their suicide risk?

There are a number of approaches to asking a patient about their potential risks around suicide, and it takes a combination of practice and confidence in your ability to be able to do this effectively. Remember that if you develop the right compassionate, non-judgemental relationship with your patient, they are very likely to speak freely and openly about their plans with you. Should this happen, it is important that you document them clearly, and verbally hand them over as part of a signposting or escalation process.

Asking about suicidal ideas

- Have you thought about ending your life?
- How often do you currently think about dying?
- Have you felt that your life is not worth living?
- Have you thought that family and friends would be better off without you?
- How long does it usually take for the thoughts to go away?

If yes to above, consider asking about suicide plans:

- Do you currently have any suicidal intent?
- Do you have specific thoughts or plans about taking your own life?
- Have you set a time or place?
- Have you done anything or taken steps to prepare to take your own life (for example, writing a suicide note or will, arranging the method, giving away possessions)?
- Are there any protective factors? (For example, some people state they could not do this to their family or children, cite religion as a protective factor or describe plans for the future. Please remember not to assume family or children are a protective factor as some people get so low and hopeless that they think they are a burden and their family are better off without them).

You will only know the level of risk and how to manage it safely if you ask questions

87

Risk Management

A key part of the mental health assessment you undertake is to identify risk factors of your patient which may predispose them to an increased risk of suicide. There are a number of tools available to help you do this, and in the UK the ambulance services should use the tool advocated in their Joint Royal Colleges Ambulance Liaison Committee (JRCALC) guidelines along with local reference guides and triage tools.

Once a patient is considered to be at risk of suicide, it is important that the right safety plans are put in place for their ongoing management as identified. In most cases, this will involve an assessment by a dedicated mental health professional. The ambulance service has many referral routes and access points to obtain clinical expert support on decision making. These may include mental health nurses in control rooms or mental health triage cars. Where necessary, please escalate to the duty line manager in your division.

Every effort should be made to encourage the patient to travel with you on an informal basis if clinically indicated. However, where you consider there is a high risk to the patient or others and the patient is refusing referral or travel, it may be necessary to consult with the GP or duty approved mental health professional (AMHP) and possibly to use the Mental Health Act. These can be accessed by the patient's GP or via the change control room. A guide to supporting decision making and scenarios under both the Mental Health Act and Mental Capacity Act is given on pages 34–43.

Procedure for practitioners working with people at risk of suicide

Dependent on the practitioner's role, this will involve:

- Compassionately assessing risk and, if necessary, escalating the case to the right agency, which could be the patient's GP or the crisis team

- Exploring safety pathways such as crisis houses, local 111/999 mental health professional lines or mental health triage cars where they are in operation (normally police or ambulance crews with mental health practitioners deployed by control rooms)

- If the patient is at high risk, demonstrating mental health crisis and refusing treatment, discuss with an on-call AMHP regarding possibility of a Mental Health Act assessment

- If the patient has already harmed themselves, for example with toxic overdose, ligature or self-harm, consider the Mental Capacity Act two-stage functional test (see page 38) along with any assessment, treatment, safeguarding or signposting proportionate to both medical and mental health risks.

Where complex, you should report any concerns or support required to normal operational escalation processes, a senior staff member or the designated safeguarding lead.

Adult patients who have been promised confidentiality by practitioners should also be informed of limits to confidentiality and understand that disclosures of suicidal intent must be shared under a duty of care.

Informed consent to share information should be sought if the child or young person is competent, unless:

- The situation is urgent and delaying in order to seek consent may result in serious harm to the young person

- Seeking consent is likely to cause serious harm to someone or to prejudice the prevention or detection of serious crime.

Professional judgement must be exercised to determine whether a child or young person is competent to consent or refuse consent to sharing information.

If consent to information sharing is refused, or can/should not be sought, information should still be shared in the following circumstances:

- There is reason to believe that not sharing information is likely to result in serious harm to the person or someone else or is likely to prejudice the prevention or detection of serious crime, and

- The risk is sufficiently great to outweigh the harm or prejudice to anyone which may be caused by the sharing, and

- There is a pressing need to share the information.

Professionals should keep parents informed and involve them in the information-sharing decision even if a child is competent or over 16. However, Gillick competence principles indicate that if a competent child wants to limit the information given to their parents or does not want them to know it at all, the child's wishes should be respected, unless the conditions for sharing without consent apply.

Where a child is not competent, a parent or person with parental responsibility should give consent unless the circumstances for sharing without consent apply.

Safety planning

Many people in distress do not know where to seek support or may be reluctant to disclose suicidal thoughts or thoughts of self-harm. Suicide cannot be accurately predicted at an individual level at a given point in time. For these reasons, a paradigm shift is required from ineffective attempts to predict risk as a means of allocating care (or not) to a universal, population-based early-intervention approach such as safety planning.

Safety planning is not a 'one-size-fits-all' approach and should be individualised and matched to the needs of the person who is in distress and the capabilities and role of the person who is supporting them. A safety plan reminds people what they can do to help themselves when distressed or during a crisis. It includes:

- Individualised strategies or activities to instil hope: Letters of hope, pictures to inspire recovery, positive memories to provide meaning

- Practical ways to stay safe: Restriction of access to means of self-harm or suicide

- Helpful and practical ways to get through tough times: Lifting and calming their mood or seeking distraction

- Reminders of emotional or social support: Including friends and family

- Specific suicide and self-harm support: Third sector, helplines, healthcare

- Directions for accessing emergency and crisis support.

Safety plans can also include ways to focus on activities of daily living such as healthy eating, suitable prescribed medication, regular sleep routine and identifying personal relapse indicators. Safety plans should also highlight the importance of self-compassion. Often hobbies, interests, pets, relaxation techniques or mindfulness support recovery. Safety plans can be co-produced by a healthcare professional but should be very much patient centred, inclusive and empowering.

4 Mental Health has developed a free website, stayingsafe.net, to ensure safety planning is accessible to people in the community, even before they seek support or emergency care. The website is co-produced by an expert reference group (people with lived experience, academics, practitioners) and features:

- Digestible step-by-step explanatory videos

- Easy-to-read, clearly written information

- A specific area for young people

- A downloadable safety plan template

- An online safety plan with pre-populated suggestions for electronic completion and storage.

Clinical tip

Take a look at the social prescribing activities described on pages 99–100 ('take 5 for mental health' section: connecting, taking notice, giving, keeping learning and being active).

Think live, love, do

Mental health protective factors often relate to **how we live, who we love and what we do**.

Consider the following questions:

- Are there any positive factors related to social prescribing that would help?

- Does the patient live alone?

- Can responsible compassionate relatives or friends support?

- Is there a care team?

- Is there a safety plan?

- What normally helps the patient manage distress?

- What structured routine or distraction skills could help?

- Is there any regular or PRN (if and when required) medication that can help?

- What social support is available?

- Are any referral routes required such as crisis team, crisis house or support workers?

- Are there any solutions or protective factors that would help?

- What inspires hope?

Services which may be available to support you with urgent and emergency mental health care

- 111, 999 or healthcare professional lines. Mental health care for all ages, with 24/7 telephone access through control rooms

- Ambulance operational triage approaches such as mental health nurses and paramedics

- Mental health training and signposting options

- Database of signposting services to support pathways and alternatives to emergency department (ED) or Section 136

- Multi-agency frequent caller mental health and social crisis care plans and pathways.

Services that can help someone who is feeling suicidal

Emergency Services and Accident and Emergency (A&E)

If someone is in immediate danger of taking their own life, consider triage cars, crisis houses, use of the Mental Health Act or use of the Mental Capacity Act if appropriate, following assessment Section 136 or ED. Ask for help through escalation processes.

Local NHS Urgent Mental Health Helpline

NHS 111, 999 or healthcare professional mental health helplines for people of all ages.

Crisis Team or Home Treatment Team

Part of NHS mental health services. They give short-term support for people having a mental health crisis, assess and manage risk and signpost where appropriate.

Community Mental Health Team (CMHT)

If a person is known to their local NHS CMHT, they may be able to access support.

Kooth

Kooth is a free online counselling and emotional well-being support service, providing young people aged 11–18 with a safe and secure means of accessing support for their emotional health and well-being needs from a professional team of qualified counsellors.

GP

Call their GP if you know who they are. A GP may be able to offer support in a crisis. If the GP surgery is closed, there will be a recorded message to tell you who to call.

Other organisations that provide a range of free support and advice

The CALM Zone
https://www.thecalmzone.net/

Connecting with People
https://www.4mentalhealth.com/?q=healthcare-front

NHS Choices
https://www.nhs.uk/mental-health/feelings-symptoms-behaviours/behaviours/help-for-suicidal-thoughts/

Rethink
https://www.rethink.org/advice-and-information/carers-hub/suicidal-thoughts-how-to-support-someone/

The Royal College of Psychiatry
https://www.rcpsych.ac.uk/healthadvice

Staying Safe
https://www.stayingsafe.net/

Time to Change
https://www.time-to-change.org.uk/mental-health-stigma

Young Minds
https://youngminds.org.uk/find-help/for-parents/

Zero Suicide Alliance
https://www.zerosuicidealliance.com/

Self-harm

Self-harm is a term that relates to intentional self-injury. Examples include, but are not limited to, cutting, scratching, intentional overdosing, hitting body parts and pulling hair. Patients who self-harm often describe it as a release for overwhelming emotional distress, a method of punishing themselves or a way to feel in control. As an ambulance clinician, it is crucial to have a compassionate, non-judgemental approach.

Often patients with a history of self-harm have a personality disorder with self-loathing and low self-esteem so any perception of feeling judged can be profound. Redirecting conversations to more productive coping strategies, de-escalation techniques, calmer background environments and existing family or professional support can be a very helpful approach. Where possible, encourage patients to talk openly and honestly about triggers and managing distress and empower them to access help.

The assessment and treatment of any injury takes priority over underlying mental health factors and should be treated like an accidental injury. There is sometimes a correlation between self-harm and suicidal ideation; however, this should not be assumed, as each patient is individual. However, not all suicidal patients have a history of self-harm and self-harm does not always indicate suicidal intent. When assessing treatment options and managing risks, do access support from the patient's family, GP and any professionals involved where appropriate. Also consider guidance under the Mental Health Act and Mental Capacity Act section to support decision making and proportionate risk management if patients refuse treatment and are high risk.

⊕ Link

For more information on where to get help for self-harm, check out the NHS website:

▶ www.nhs.uk/conditions/self-harm

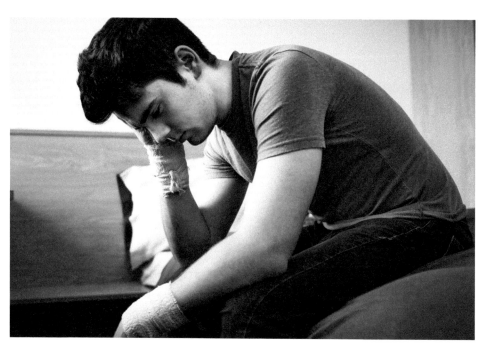

Part 5

Support in the Ambulance Service

This section includes:

- **The Mental Health Continuum**

- **Resilience and Bounceability**

- **Social Prescribing**

- **Where to Find Support**

- **A Framework for Staff Mental Health**

The Mental Health Continuum

What is the mental health continuum?

The concept of a mental health continuum was briefly covered earlier in the workbook, on page 10. The mental health continuum is a tool which helps us to think about our well-being and what actions we can take to improve it. The mental health continuum helps us to identify where our mental health is now.

Mental health is not an 'all or nothing' concept – it can change often. Mental health is affected by lots of things, such as work, home life, bereavement, ill health and more. Even positive things can affect our mental health, like the pressure after getting a promotion or the stress of a house move. We will all experience difficulties at some point during our life. A continuum is used to show that we can move between the different states of well-being: thriving, surviving, struggling and crisis.

How do I use the mental health continuum?

You can use the mental health continuum alone or with others.

Use the tool to answer the question 'Thinking about your well-being in the past week, do you feel…'.

By looking at the different statements you can assess your well-being. You do not have to agree with every statement to fit into a category. For example, you may be thriving socially despite feeling you are in crisis overall.

When you have thought about where you fit best, take action using the coloured boxes at the bottom of the tool.

Who is the mental health continuum for?

The mental health continuum can be used by anyone.

Examples

Shift check-in
Mohammed and Claire are working together. At the start of the shift they check in to see where they are on the continuum. Mohammed is feeling green. Claire is feeling orange. Knowing how each other are doing helps them to work together. They talk about how Claire has had a difficult run of shifts, affecting her sleep.

Appraisal
Zara line manages Paul. They meet to discuss Paul's appraisal. Zara uses the mental health continuum to ask Paul how he is doing. Paul is able to reflect on his well-being. He has been thriving socially and doing well physically but notices that he can be impatient and struggle with stress. They agree a plan for him to engage in peer support.

Return to work
Phil is returning to work after time off due to illness. Phil uses the continuum to think about how they are feeling. Phil notices that they have been struggling more than they realised. Phil decides to speak to their line manager. Together they decide Phil should talk to their GP and Phil makes a note to arrange an appointment at the end of the shift.

How are you really doing?
Thinking about your well-being in the past week, do you feel...

	THRIVING	SURVIVING	STRUGGLING	IN CRISIS	
EMOTIONAL	In good spirits with usual ups and downs Positive about life most of the time	Sometimes irritable, impatient, nervous or sad Positive about life some of the time	Often impatient, nervous or sad Coping with the stresses of daily life is often hard	Angry, anxious, hopeless or always sad Overwhelmed by the stresses of daily life	**EMOTIONAL**
PSYCHOLOGICAL	Able to cope with the stresses of daily life A sense of purpose in life most of the time No thoughts of suicide or fleeting thoughts of suicide	Mostly able to cope with stresses of daily life Unsure about your sense of purpose in life Some thoughts of suicide with no plans to act on these	Negative about life some of the time Disinterest or that life lacks purpose sometimes Thoughts of suicide, including some planning related to these	Negative about life most of the time Disinterested or that life lacks purpose most of the time Thoughts of suicide and active plans to act on these	**PSYCHOLOGICAL**
SOCIAL	Able to take part in social activities or hobbies as much as you'd like Supported by family, friends and colleagues	Able to take part in social activities or hobbies sometimes Somewhat supported by family, friends and colleagues	Rarely able to take part in social activities or hobbies Disconnect from family, friends and colleagues	Mostly unable to take part in social activities or hobbies Withdrawn from or avoiding family, friends and colleagues	**SOCIAL**
PHYSICAL	Physically well for you Considering your shift pattern, you are able to get quality rest and sleep Able to do as much physical activity as you'd like within your usual capability	Mostly physically well Aside from any disruption caused by shift pattern, your sleep is disturbed sometimes Able to do some physical activity within your usual capability	Sometimes physically unwell Aside from any disruption caused by shift pattern, it is difficult getting quality rest and sleep Unable to do much physical activity within your usual capability	Physically unwell for you Aside from any disruption caused by shift pattern, you are unable to get quality rest and sleep Unable to do any physical activity within your usual capability	**PHYSICAL**
ADDICTION	You have not used addictive behaviours (e.g. alcohol, substances, gambling, food) to cope	You have rarely used addictive behaviours (e.g. alcohol, substances, gambling, food) to cope	You have sometimes used addictive behaviours (e.g. alcohol, substances, gambling, food) to cope	You have frequently used addictive behaviours (e.g. alcohol, substances, gambling, food) to cope	**ADDICTION**

⬅ We all experience times when we struggle or reach crisis. It is ok to not be ok.
Your loved ones, employer and professionals can help. ➡

MAINTAIN YOUR WELL-BEING	**PROMOTE YOUR WELL-BEING**	**FOCUS ON YOUR WELL-BEING**	**PRIORITISE YOUR WELL-BEING**
Connect with others Be physically active Learn new skills Give Be present in the moment	Actively engage in coping techniques and self-care Engage in peer support and clinical supervision Reflective practice – what are your support needs?	Connect with your line manager, employee support services or GP Talk about how you are feeling Consider trying a new coping technique	Prioritise asking for support from employee support services, the Ambulance Staff Charity, your GP or in an emergency 999 (you're a person too, 999 is there for you)

© Dr Jaimee Wylam, Speciality Registrar in Public Health in partnership with task and finish expert reference group

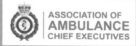
ASSOCIATION OF
AMBULANCE
CHIEF EXECUTIVES

Visit
bluelighttogether.org.uk ➡

Resilience and Bounceability

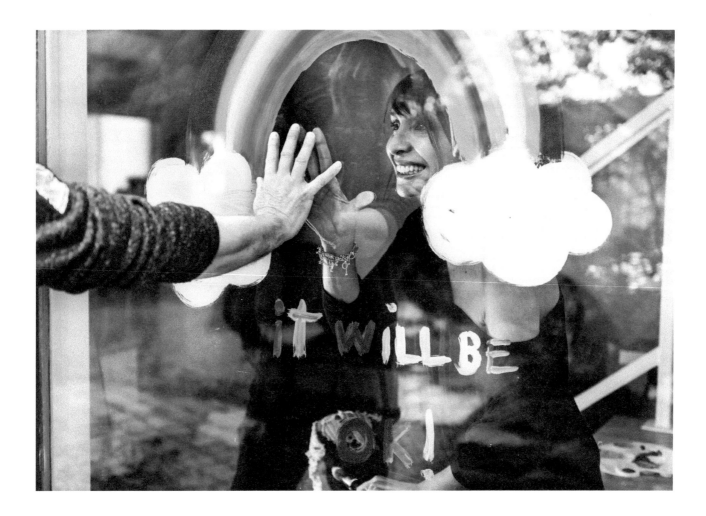

Within the ambulance service, it is in our remit to ensure timely access to high-quality care for the mental health of our people, our patients and our partnerships. It is important to remember that mental health is not just about the absence of illness. Like physical health, there are a number of positive steps we can take to maintain and improve our levels of mental well-being or resilience.

Resilience

Resilience can be seen as our capacity to cope with life setbacks, changes to circumstances, pressures, demands and normal daily activities.

It is our drive and desire to succeed and bounce back from stress and adversity. We are all unique and cope differently with stress and pressure. Over time, if stress is not recognised or managed it can have an impact on our resilience and day-to-day functioning. Stress also activates the threat and self-protection part of our brain. This means we tend to focus much more on worries or things that are difficult to resolve. We then reduce the time we spend on drive and desire and compassion and self-soothing. By engaging the drive and desire and compassion and self-soothing parts of our brain, we are providing space to refresh and put things into perspective.

Bounceability

Resilience can be seen as our ability to bounce back from life events and pressures. A good analogy would be to see 'bounceability' as a beach ball. When the beach ball is fully inflated, it bounces back from day-to-day challenges. If we are drained and overcome with a combination of work pressures, relationship pressures or financial pressures, this can all impact our bounceability by slowly losing air from the beach ball. Suddenly, and often without notice, this can impact our ability to bounce back from life stressors. In order to regain resilience, we need to re-inflate our beach ball by objectively detaching from the worries and excessive ruminations. By being self-compassionate and finding ways to switch off, we can refresh and refocus on solutions to life stressors. It is important to remember that compassion starts from within and that if there is nothing left in the tank, there is nothing left to give.

⊕ Link

A valuable website on mental health support and awareness is:

▶ www.nhs.uk/oneyou/every-mind-matters

Social Prescribing

Like physical health, we all have to look after our mental health, and mental health is not just the absence of illness. Social prescribing is a term used commonly in primary care, and is related to referral routes and ways to promote resilience and mental well-being or early intervention to reduce the risk of mental state deterioration. There are five key components to social prescribing, as outlined below.

Take 5 for mental health

The Public Health Agency recommends five simple steps to improve our mental health and well-being (Public Health Agency, 2020).

1. Connect

Interacting with others. Are you isolating yourself more or reflective, self aware and engaging? Think about relationships with family, friends and work colleagues. Do you still have the same level of contact and support with them? Are the interactions positive and helpful? If not, what would need to change?

2. Take notice

Taking time to be aware of our surroundings and being present in the moment. Not being distracted or multitasking (be present in the experience). Think about examples of slowing down thoughts, relaxation and mindfulness. Abdominal breathing exercises and deep muscular exercise can be a very productive way of managing stress and switching off.

3. Give

Taking time to show compassion for others and creating a 'currency of kindness'. Consider the concept that behaviour breeds behaviour. When we demonstrate courtesy, dignity and respect we are more likely to receive this back. If we are stressed, rude or abrupt we are more likely to receive defensiveness. Think about random acts of kindness when you intervened to brighten someone's mood or when someone did this for you (for example, holding a door open for someone, allowing someone out in a traffic queue, helping an someone get something from the top shelf in a shop). Sometimes simple acts that take little effort from us can have a powerful impact on people's lives. People are innately social beings and we should try to support each other if we feel lonely or isolated.

4. Keep learning

When it comes to problem solving and solution-focused approaches, think about new ways of learning or tackling a difficult-to-resolve situation. If something is playing on your mind, seek coaching support or supervision from a trusted colleague or friend. They may be able to offer a different perspective that helps unblock a challenge or
fresh ideas. Hobbies and interests such crosswords or sudoku, reading, music, DIY, art and design, volunteering in groups and many others help with our sense of enjoyment and trying new things.

5. Regular exercise and healthy living

Regular exercise helps us both physically and mentally. Examples such as running, bike rides,

🌐 Link

Further information on social prescribing can be found on the NHS website:

▶ https://www.england.nhs.uk/personalisedcare/social-prescribing/

team sports, swimming or brisk walks produce feel-good chemicals and emotions such as endorphins and oxytocin. These are natural ways to help lift your mood and switch off. Regular exercise also provides space to think and is a useful distraction from things that can play on our minds.

Remember, compassion starts from within. If we do not have self-compassion or are not in a good place emotionally, it can be difficult to be compassionate to others. As mentioned earlier, we are all unique and have unique strengths. We are also often our own worst critics! By reflecting on and acknowledging vulnerabilities, we can reach a greater level of acceptance and understanding of our strengths and vulnerabilities. Not everyone will enjoy or do the same things when it comes to exercise, hobbies or interests. It is useful though to reflect on two or three different options within the 'take 5 for mental health' framework. This builds a sense of purpose, structure and distraction in order to have the right work–life balance.

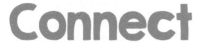
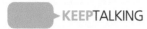
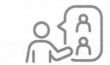

Talk & listen, Be there, Feel connected

Your time, Your words, Your presence

Take Notice

Remember the simple things that give you joy

Take 5 For mental health

Keep Learning

Embrace new experiences, see opportunities, surprise yourself

Be Active

Do what you can, enjoy what you do, move your mood

Where to Find Support

Like physical health, we all have to look after our mental health and we can all take positive steps to manage stress and improve resilience through awareness and reflection.

Unlike physical health problems, it can be difficult to see or recognise a mental health problem, even for the person experiencing it. We do often, however, (if we take notice) see a change in someone's behaviour over time. Anxiety, stress and depression are the most common forms of mental health conditions experienced by ambulance service staff. Unlike physical health problems, anxiety, stress and depression can often build up over time and without noticing.

If unrecognised and untreated, this can have an impact on our activities of daily living and functioning to a point where it may become a clinical condition. Another main potential area of focus on mental health conditions in supporting ambulance service personnel is post-traumatic stress disorder (PTSD). A qualified doctor would need to diagnose PTSD and if PTSD is suspected a referral to Occupational Health should be arranged.

Support services in the ambulance service

Our people are the most valuable asset we have and it is important to acknowledge the work that they do on a day-to-day basis. It is also essential that we have supporting mechanisms in place to help them if and when they are in need. Within the ambulance service, we have the following supporting mechanisms in place:

- Trauma Risk Management (TRiM)
- Peer support workers
- Occupational health and employee assistance programmes.

Trauma Risk Management (TRiM)

Trauma Risk Management (TRiM) is a trauma-focused peer-support system based on assessing employees' functioning after traumatic events, and is commonly used in the ambulance sector (marchonstress.com). It provides support and signposting for staff who require it.

TRiM provides a structured process to ensure there and trained staff providing initial assessment to ambulance employees who may have experienced a traumatic event which could be impacting day to day functioning or thought processes. Acknowledging the complexity of the role that our frontline clinicians undertake, it is important to recognise that TRiM is not a treatment for PTSD but a process to assess any potential signs of PTSD for onward referral where appropriate. TRiM as a process can either be suggested following recognition of a potentially traumatic incident by a colleague or manager, or can be self-referred to your TRiM co-ordinator where available following internal processes. TRiM is not a treatment process but a risk assessment of any requirement for treatment. TRiM can recommend a referral to Occupational Health to be assessed by a qualified mental health practitioner for counselling and support. This could include trauma-informed cognitive behaviour therapy (CBT) or eye movement desensitisation and reprocessing (EMDR) along with a range of other treatment options.

Peer support workers

Your employer may have a well-being peer support network. This often involves a number of volunteers from within the service who have been taken on additional training in mental health awareness to provide a supportive network allowing anyone experiencing difficulties to discuss their feelings in a compassionate and supportive way. Examples of training within peer support networks include mental health first aid (MHFA) and psychological first aid (PFA).

Although supportive peer workers are not counsellors, they can provide a framework for compassionate listening. They can also find and provide practical assistance to find solutions to problems, including signposting to other support mechanisms where appropriate.

They should actively listen to provide confidential support and a compassionate approach to all members of staff. There should also be a clear support, supervision and escalation process within each organisation to provide governance.

Occupational health support

Your employer should have a range of personal and professional resources to support resilience and occupational mental health support. They should offer confidential line management and a personal support service that is available 24/7.

A Framework for Staff Mental Health

Key principles of mental health support

Given the pressures of the ambulance service, global uncertainties and the impact of COVID-19, your employer should prioritise mental health awareness and support in the workplace. This should cover the importance of close collaboration between clinical occupational mental health support and any wider wellbeing team. A structured framework should be agreed on to improve mental health and psychological safety in the workplace.

This sits within four key principles; promotion, prevention, intervention and recovery. These are outlined in more detail in the following pages. Please remember the importance of a non-judgemental approach, compassion, dignity, respect and trust around contact with any colleague experiencing a mental health or social care crisis. A solution-focused approach and good listening skills help de-escalation, managing distress and resilience.

Promotion, prevention, intervention and recovery

Staff programmes for mental health should focus on:

Promotion

Improving recognition and normalising mental health awareness in the workplace. This involves tackling stigma and taboos related to mental health which could prevent or delay access if staff feel judged. The ambulance service has produced a number of resources related to this, such as the AACE 'Ambulance Wellbeing Resources' (https://aace.org.uk/resources/resource-category/ambulance-wellbeing/) and 'Supporting Ambulance Staff on Mental Health and Wellbeing' webpages (https://aace.org.uk/mentalhealthandwellbeing/).

Prevention

There are various models of first-contact mental health support within the workplace. Some ambulance service trusts include training courses for staff, such as Mental Health First Aid (MHFA) or Psychological First Aid (PFA), to develop a peer support programme. These can act as a first point of contact for compassionate conversations and signposting advice around staff mental health.

These programmes should be done in partnership with the health and wellbeing, leadership and education teams, so that ambulance services can continue to build the right information, workshops and awareness sessions though induction, manager awareness sessions and CPD sessions.

Intervention

It is crucial to have timely access to high-quality care in a mental health crisis. The ambulance service will continue to grow and develop their occupational health offer specific to mental health. This will include an options appraisal on access to specialist mental health either through referral within Occupational Health or via relevant NHS provision. A red flag escalation process for staff at risk to themselves or others related to mental health will be enhanced.

Recovery

Like physical health, people who are living with or have recovered from a mental health condition should have all reasonable adjustments and support plans in place to maximise potential for a sustained recovery. Trusts should continue to encourage, grow and develop personalised well-being recovery action plans. This will help identify triggers and the importance of access to support to prevent a relapse where possible.

Signposting

Useful video links

I had a black dog. His name was depression
(As seen in 'Key conditions encountered in prehospital care', page 54)
https://youtu.be/XiCrniLQGYc

Transport for London: Share the Road, M&C Saatchi London
(As seen in 'Initial assessment of a patient with a mental illness', page 26)
www.youtube.com/watch?v=ObTkJpVJgs8

Mind Blue Light Programme
https://www.mind.org.uk/news-campaigns/campaigns/blue-light-programme/

Drew Dudley, TEDx Talks 'Leading with Lollipops'
https://www.youtube.com/watch?v=hVCBrkrFrBE

Websites and apps

4 Mental Health
https://www.4mentalhealth.com/

Campaign Against Living Miserably
https://www.thecalmzone.net/

Every Mind Matters
https://www.nhs.uk/every-mind-matters/

JAAQ (Just Ask A Question)
https://jaaq.co.uk/about-jaaq/

Mental Health First Aid (MHFA)
https://mhfaengland.org/

NHS – Help for Suicidal Thoughts
https://www.nhs.uk/mental-health/feelings-symptoms-behaviours/behaviours/help-for-suicidal-thoughts/

NHS – Social Prescribing
https://www.england.nhs.uk/personalisedcare/social-prescribing/

Papyrus
https://www.papyrus-uk.org/

Psychological First Aid (PFA)
https://www.futurelearn.com/courses/psychological-first-aid-for-children-and-young-people

Rethink Mental Illness – Suicidal Thoughts: How to Support Someone
https://www.rethink.org/advice-and-information/carers-hub/suicidal-thoughts-how-to-support-someone/

Royal College of Psychiatry – Mental Health
https://www.rcpsych.ac.uk/mental-health

Samaritans
https://www.samaritans.org/

Staying Safe from Suicidal Thoughts
https://www.stayingsafe.net/

Suicide Bereavement UK
https://suicidebereavementuk.com/

Suicide First Aid (SFA)
https://www.suicidefirstaid.uk/

Time to Change – Mental Health & Stigma
https://www.time-to-change.org.uk/mental-health-stigma

Zero Suicide Alliance
https://www.zerosuicidealliance.com/

Young Minds
https://www.youngminds.org.uk/

Glossary

AMHP: Approved mental health professional who is responsible for co-ordinating a Mental Health Act assessment

AMPDS: Advanced Medical Priority Dispatch System

AOT: Assertive outreach team. Specialist mental health team offering intensive support for patients who have enduring mental health problems, are treatment resistive and require intensive community support

CRT: Crisis resolution team: Community assessment and intensive home treatment team offering short-term **intensive** support following a crisis as an alternative to inpatient admission

Early intervention psychosis team: Specialist team supporting patients who first present with an enduring psychotic episode

HBPOS: Health-based place of safety for patients detained under Section 136 normally connected to the local mental health hospital

MHA: Mental Health Act. A formal legal process to assess a patient deemed to be at significant risk to themselves or others who is refusing treatment, or voluntary admission where there is suspected evidence of a treatable mental illness

POS: Place of safety. Any specific location nominated by the locality area or with the permission of the patient and home owner. Police cells should be a last resort as a place of safety and should never be used for children detained under Section 136

References

4AT Rapid Clinical Test for Delirium. n.d. Available at: https://www.the4at.com/.

Alcohol Change UK, 2021. Alcohol statistics. Available at: https://alcoholchange.org.uk/alcohol-facts/fact-sheets/alcohol-statistics.

Alcohol Change UK, n.d. Alcohol and inequalities. Policy insights. Available at: https://alcoholchange.org.uk/policy/policy-insights/alcohol-and-inequalities.

Alzheimer's Society, 2021. Young-onset dementia. Available at: https://www.alzheimers.org.uk/about-dementia/types-dementia/young-onset-dementia.

Association of Ambulance Chief Executives, n.d. Resource Category: Ambulance Wellbeing. Available at: https://aace.org.uk/resources/resource-category/ambulance-wellbeing/.

Association of Ambulance Chief Executives, n.d. Supporting Ambulance Staff on Mental Health and Wellbeing. Available at: https://aace.org.uk/mentalhealthandwellbeing/.

Autistica, n.d. Suicide and autism. Available at: https://www.autistica.org.uk/what-is-autism/signs-and-symptoms/suicide-and-autism.

Bishop-Fitzpatrick, L., and Kind, A.J.H. 2017. A Scoping Review of Health Disparities in Autism Spectrum Disorder. *Journal of Autism and Developmental Disorders*, 47: 3380–3391.

Davies, T. and Craig, T.K.J. 1998. *ABC of Mental Health*. London: BMJ Books.

Delamere, 2021. The UK Drug and Alcohol Use Survey 2021. Available at: https://delamere.com/blog/the-uk-drug-and-alcohol-use-survey-2021#overview.

Dementia UK, 2021. What is dementia? Available at: https://www.dementiauk.org/about-dementia/dementia-information/what-is-dementia/.

Department for Constitutional Affairs (DCA), 2007. Mental Capacity Act 2005: Code of Practice. London: The Stationery Office.

Department of Health, 2015. Mental Health Act 1983: Code of Practice. Norwich: The Stationery Office. Available at: https://www.gov.uk/government/publications/code-of-practice-mental-health-act-1983.

Department of Health & Social Care, 2021. Liberty Protection Safeguards: what they are. Available at: https://www.gov.uk/government/publications/liberty-protection-safeguards-factsheets/liberty-protection-safeguards-what-they-are.

Doherty, M, et al. 2022. Barriers to healthcare and self-reported adverse outcomes for autistic adults: a cross-sectional study. *BMJ Open*, 12: e056904.

Engel, G. 1977. The need for a new medical model: A challenge for biomedical science. *Science*, 196: 126–129.

Ewing, J. 1984. Detecting Alcoholism: The CAGE Questionnaire. *Journal of the American Medical Association*, 252(14): 1905–1907.

Foundation for People with Learning Disabilities, 2021. Learning disability statistics. Available at: https://www.learningdisabilities.org.uk/learning-disabilities/help-information/learning-disability-statistics-.

Foundation for People with Learning Disabilities, 2022. Learning disability statistics: Autism. Available at: https://www.learningdisabilities.org.uk/learning-disabilities/help-information/statistics/learning-disability-statistics-/187690.

Goleman, D. 1996. *Emotional Intelligence: Why It Can Matter More than IQ*. London: Bloomsbury Publishing.

Guan, J., and Li, G. 2017. Injury Mortality in Individuals With Autism. *American Journal of Public Health*, 107(5): 791–793.

Health and Social Care Information Centre (HSCIC), 2009. Adult psychiatric morbidity in England - 2007, Results of a household survey. Available at: https://digital.nhs.uk/data-and-information/publications/statistical/adult-psychiatric-morbidity-survey/adult-psychiatric-morbidity-in-england-2007-results-of-a-household-survey.

Healthcare Quality Improvement Partnership (HQIP), 2021. National confidential inquiry into suicide and safety in mental health – Annual report 2020. Available at: https://www.hqip.org.uk/resource/suicide-safety-mental-health-report-2020/#.YgP19ljP1pQ.

Hosking, F. J., Carey, I. M., Shah, S. M. et al. 2016. Mortality among adults with intellectual disability in England: Comparisons with the general population. *American Journal of Public Health*, 106: 1483–1490.

Iacoboni, M. 2008. *Mirroring People: The New Science of How We Connect with Others*. New York, NY: Picador.

Loomes, R., Hull, L. and Mandy, W. P. L. 2017. What is the male-to-female ratio in autism spectrum disorder? A systematic review and meta-analysis. *Journal of the American Academy of Child and Adolescent Psychiatry*, 56(6): 466–474. DOI: 10.1016/j.jaac.2017.03.013.

Mencap, 2007. Death by indifference: Following up the Treat me right! report. Available at: https://www.mencap.org.uk/sites/default/files/2016-06/DBIreport.pdf.

Mencap, 2018. Communicating with people with a learning disability. Available at: https://www.mencap.org.uk/sites/default/files/2016-12/Communicating%20with%20people_updated%20%281%29.pdf.

Mencap, n.d. Diagnosis. Available at: https://www.mencap.org.uk/advice-and-support/diagnosis.

Mental Health First Aid England, 2020. Mental health statistics. Available at: https://mhfaengland.org/mhfa-centre/research-and-evaluation/mental-health-statistics/.

Mental Health Foundation (MHF), 2021a. Mental health statistics. Available at: https://www.mentalhealth.org.uk/statistics.

Mental Health Foundation (MHF), 2021b. Stigma and discrimination. Available at: https://www.mentalhealth.org.uk/a-to-z/s/stigma-and-discrimination.

Mind, 2017. Mental health facts and statistics. Available at: https://www.mind.org.uk/media-a/2958/statistics-facts-2017.pdf.

Mind, 2020. Mental health facts and statistics. Available at: https://www.mind.org.uk/information-support/types-of-mental-health-problems/statistics-and-facts-about-mental-health/how-common-are-mental-health-problems/.

Mind, 2021. Anxiety and panic attacks. Available at: https://www.mind.org.uk/information-support/types-of-mental-health-problems/anxiety-and-panic-attacks/.

NHS England, 2016. The five year forward view for mental health. Available at: https://www.england.nhs.uk/wp-content/uploads/2016/02/Mental-Health-Taskforce-FYFV-final.pdf.

NHS, 2019a. Clinical depression. Available at: https://www.nhs.uk/mental-health/conditions/clinical-depression/.

NHS, 2019b. Psychosis. Available at: https://www.nhs.uk/mental-health/conditions/psychosis/.

NHS, 2019c. Schizophrenia. Available at: https://www.nhs.uk/mental-health/conditions/schizophrenia/.

NHS, 2021. Eating disorders. Available at: https://www.nhs.uk/mental-health/feelings-symptoms-behaviours/behaviours/eating-disorders/.

NHS, 2022. Learning disabilities. Available at: https://www.nhs.uk/conditions/learning-disabilities/.

NHS Digital, 2020a. Autism Waiting Time Statistics – Quarter 1 to Quarter 4 2019–20 and Quarter 1 (April to June) 2020–21. Available at: https://digital.nhs.uk/data-and-information/publications/statistical/autism-statistics/q1-april-to-june-2020-21/data-quality-copy.

NHS Digital, 2020b. Health and care of people with learning disabilities, experimental statistics: 2018 to 2019 [PAS]. Available at: https://digital.nhs.uk/data-and-information/publications/statistical/health-and-care-of-people-with-learning-disabilities/experimental-statistics-2018-to-2019.

NHS England, 2021. Crisis and acute mental health services. Available at: www.england.nhs.uk/mental-health/adults/crisis-and-acute-care/.

NICE, 2009. Borderline personality disorder: Recognition and management [CG78]. Available at: https://www.nice.org.uk/guidance/cg78.

NICE, 2014. Anxiety disorders [QS53], Pharmalogical treatment. Available at: https://www.nice.org.uk/guidance/qs53/chapter/quality-statement-3-pharmacological-treatment.

NICE, 2018. Post-traumatic stress disorder [NG116]. Available at: https://www.nice.org.uk/guidance/ng116/.

NICE, 2022. British National Formulary (BNF), Clozapine. Available at: https://bnf.nice.org.uk/drug/clozapine.html.

NWAS, n.d. BASIC STEPS Mental health assessment. Available at: https://www.nwyhelearning.nhs.uk/elearning/northwest/NWAS/MENTAL_HEALTH/BasicSteps_2021_Update/story.html.

Oates, L. 2019. #ProjectA mental health basic step tool: Sir Peter Carr Award finalists. *NHS Horizons*. Available at: https://nhshorizons.

passle.net/post/102ftd6/projecta-mental-health-basic-step-tool-sir-peter-carr-award-finalists#:~:text=The%20Mental%20Health%20BASIC%20STEP,%2C%20Emotional%20State%2C%20Plan).

Office for National Statistics (ONS), 2020. Suicides in England and Wales: 2019 registrations. Available at: https://www.ons.gov.uk/peoplepopulationandcommunity/birthsdeathsandmarriages/deaths/bulletins/suicidesintheunitedkingdom/2019registrations.

Public Health Agency, 2020. Take 5 steps to wellbeing. Available at: https://www.publichealth.hscni.net/publications/take-5-steps-wellbeing-english-and-11-translations.

Rickard, W. and Donkin, A. 2018. A fair, supportive society: Summary report. Available at: https://www.instituteofhealthequity.org/resources-reports/a-fair-supportive-society-summary-report.

Royal College of Psychiatrists, 2015. Personality disorder. Available at: https://www.rcpsych.ac.uk/mental-health/problems-disorders/personality-disorder.

Royal College of Psychiatrists, 2021. Record number of children and young people referred to mental health services as pandemic takes its toll. Available at: https://www.rcpsych.ac.uk/news-and-features/latest-news/detail/2021/09/23/record-number-of-children-and-young-people-referred-to-mental-health-services-as-pandemic-takes-its-toll

R (Sessay) v South London and Maudsley NHS Foundation Trust [2011] EWHC 2617.

UK Government, 2020. Autism. POSTnote 612. Available at: https://researchbriefings.files.parliament.uk/documents/POST-PN-0612/POST-PN-0612.pdf.

World Health Organization (WHO), 2021. Depression. Available at: https://www.who.int/news-room/fact-sheets/detail/depression.

Index